The Band of the Year

Everyone cherishes some memory that stands out from the rest and for me it is the night of Friday 18th April, 1969. The venue was the Lyceum Ballroom in London, I had just won the prestigious Carl-Alan award and I was certain that I had reached the high-spot of my career. I had been nominated in the previous two years - always the bridesmaid, never the bride, so to speak - but in 1969 the Phil Moss Band was voted the most outstanding resident band of the year.

I remember sitting in the rest room of the Lyceum, the flagship of Mecca's ballrooms, consciously relaxing and clutching the statuette which had just been presented to me

by film star Jack Hawkins. In the distance I could hear the dance music being played by the Ray McVey Band, which had taken over whilst my own seventeen-piece outfit was resting after a gruelling forty-five-minute television show.

It's a strange thing, but when one hears music from a distance, the treble sounds of the front line tend to fade out, although the pounding of the rhythm still comes through. My thoughts drifted to the time when my parents bought me my first second-hand trumpet and dinner suit for £3 - not a bad investment, as it transpired!

I was still aware of the sound of the drums next door, but now the beat seemed to be

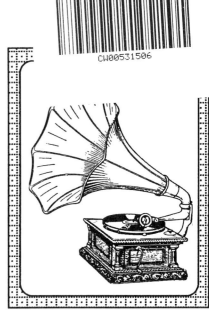

The wind-up gramophone of the 1920s - an early memory

coming from a lot further away. Some two hundred miles away, in fact, and years back in time, where a young boy was banging away on a large drum in Newton Heath, Manchester. The drum had been bought to keep me occupied, but the neighbours weren't in sympathy with the idea and it wasn't very long before the thing did a permanent vanishing trick.

With the drum just a memory, I became obsessed with the sounds of our local brass bands - the Failsworth District Band and the Culcheth Top Hat Band. The latter was the only one in the country distinguished by its sartorial headgear. I saw the band for the first time in the Whit Week walks and followed it for miles, eventually getting hopelessly lost. I was rescued by a very large and friendly policeman, who escorted me to the nearest police station - to be called for later. The police were there to be seen in those days. It was the era of cobbled streets and horse and cart vendors; when men doffed their caps and went home with unopened wage packets - 'nowt tekken out'.

The next musical event in my memory was the arrival at home of a gramophone. It was a square box effort with a very large horn and an interior spring

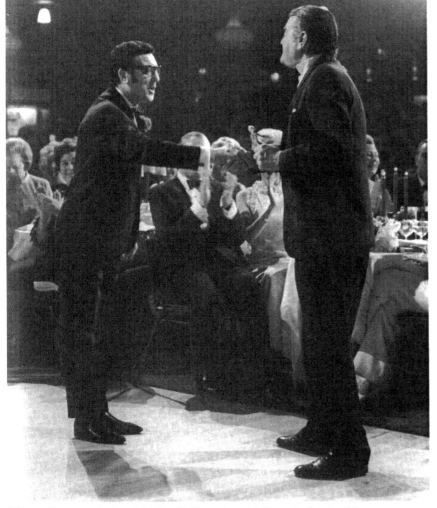

The author receiving his Carl-Alan Award from Jack Hawkins

which had to be wound up for each record played. I played the half-dozen records incessantly, until one day the overworked spring gave up the ghost and the machine ground to a terminal halt.

It was unanimously decided that a mouth-organ might be a safer and cheaper outlet for my musical ambitions. My first one was called 'The Bandmaster'. Prophetic? It had been made in Germany by Hohner, was priced one shilling (5p today) and I played it at every opportunity. I actually progressed to such an extent that I started to enter and win local talent contests. My new idol was then Larry Adler - 'Mouth Almighty' - who was raising the status of the mouth organ from that of a toy to being accepted as a respected instrument in large American orchestras.

To avoid getting involved with a mind-numbing autobiography, I'm going to glide smartly through succeeding stages in my career, albeit returning to events from time to time. I joined the local bugle band, went on to play in brass bands in the

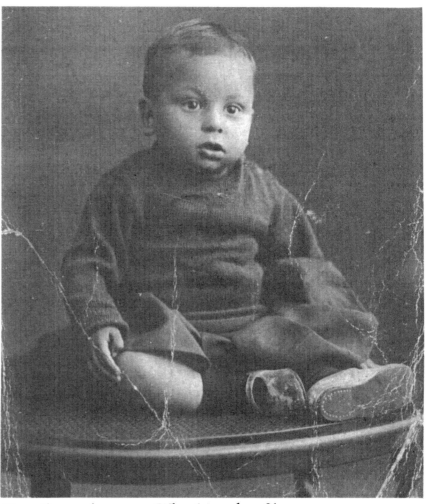

The author aged one year. 'Where's my drum?'

parks on Sunday afternoons, then progressed from playing the cornet to the trumpet in local dance bands. From there it was straight into the world of ballrooms, which were my second home for some fifty years.

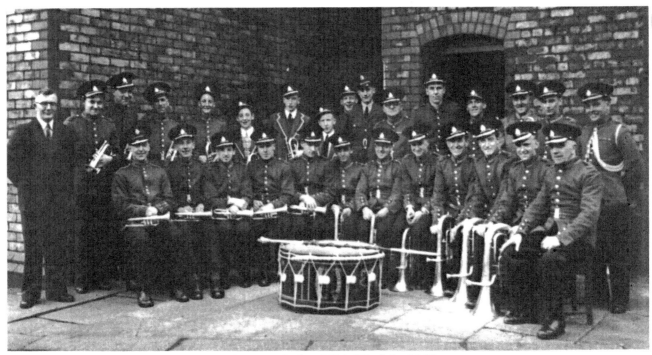

Failsworth and District Brass Band, photographed at Whit Week in 1949

Oh, How They Danced!

It is safe to say that for decades ballroom dancing was one of the most popular and pleasurable pastimes in the Western World. Dancing is probably one of the most natural instincts known to man, next to eating and drinking, and the ballroom presented a convenient and widely available opportunity for the opposite sexes to meet.

'Boy meets girl' is as old as the universe itself and the ability to dance was considered to be a great social asset; a sure passport to meeting new friends and making romantic attachments. Further on in these pages we shall meet some of the personalities of the Manchester ballroom scene and consider the rise and fall in popularity of the big bands and their venues. We can applaud some of the survivors and encourage the newcomers who will take music into the next century. Music and dancing are still alive and in the hands of young and enthusiastic performers, so The Song is definitely not ended and the Melody *will* linger on!

Manchester's Local Ballrooms

Manchester has always been one of the busiest centres of the ballroom dancing industry. When we recall the various ballrooms of our city, we are inclined to think first of the larger venues, such as the Belle Vue Elizabethan Hall or the Ritz in the city centre, but there were many others in the surrounding districts and they all thrived in the boom of the post-war years. They also provided a good source of income for the well-known professional teachers and demonstrators.

The ballroom fraternity will

recall the exhibitions given by Cyril Farmer and Adele Roscoe, and Sid Perkins and Edna Duffield. Other familiar names were Len Scrivener and Nellie Dougan; Eric Hancox (the Major) and Betty Wych. Firm favourites were Sonny Binnick and Sally Brock, Charles and Joan Thiebalt, Wally Fryer and Violet Barnes, Harry Smith-Hampshire and Doreen Casey. Wally Green was a regular feature with his partner, Mrs Adams.

Tommy Rogers and Hilda Lamont opened their dance academy in Oxford Road, and of course there was the ever-present Finnigan's Dance Academy with Frank and Joan Gibson. The Rowsley Street Co-op was another popular venue, boasting a beautiful staircase that led up to the ballroom. Friday night was the most popular night of the week at Shorrocks' in Brunswick Street,

Chorlton-on-Medlock, with an admission fee of a shilling.

Albert Cowan (known as the 'Grand Old Man of Dancing') had his twin ballroom academy in Raby Street, Moss Side. He would instruct all the lady pupils in one hall and his wife taught all the males in the other. Albert always said he could never remember faces, as he always danced with his hands on his partners' shoulders and his eyes on their feet. When the packed tramcars reached Raby Street the guard would shout, 'All out for Cowan's!' The tram would empty of passengers, all carrying their dance slippers wrapped in brown paper. Again, admission was a 'bob' (a shilling), with an extra penny for cloakroom fee.

One of the first ballrooms in which I played was Winifred's in All Saints. I remember when I saw the advert - 'Trumpet player wanted for band at Winifred's Ballroom' - I broke all existing records getting

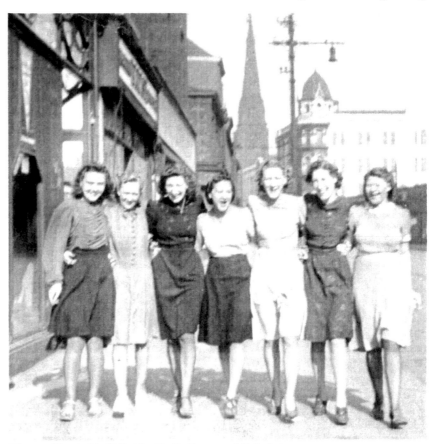

The staff outside Winifred's Ballroom, All Saints

myself down to the place. I had imagined that the ballroom itself had been christened 'Winifred's' and wasn't prepared for the interview that followed. Instead of being quizzed by some experienced bandleader, I was introduced to Winifred herself, the daughter of the famous footballer Billy Meredith, who played for both Manchester United and Manchester City. She was a glamorous young lady with attractive features, skilfully applied make-up and a dark, well groomed head of hair. All of which made me forget for a moment the reason for my visit. I remember she looked me up and down carefully, as if measuring me for a band uniform, then there was a quick, businesslike conversation which brought me back down to earth.

The following evening I played with the house band, was given the job and stayed at Winifred's for several months before moving on. I was always motivated by the urge to climb another rung of the ladder!

Mr Bill Hall and his brother

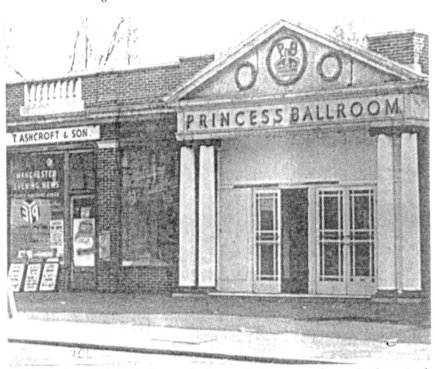

The Chorlton Palais de Danse Princess Ballroom, a favourite haunt of ballroom dancers in South Manchester

Jack were probably the most ambitious of entrepreneurs in Manchester in the thirties and forties. They promoted several halls: the Lido on Ashton Old Road, the Rex Ballroom in Stockport, the High Street, Harpurhey and Moston Baths Ballrooms, and later (1938) the noted Burton Ballroom at Blackpool. Six ventures in all, and I played in each of them over the years.

After I left Winifred's Ballroom in 1937 I started at the Lido - a glamorous name which did much to hide the lack of glamour in its location at the corner of Claribel Street. I joined

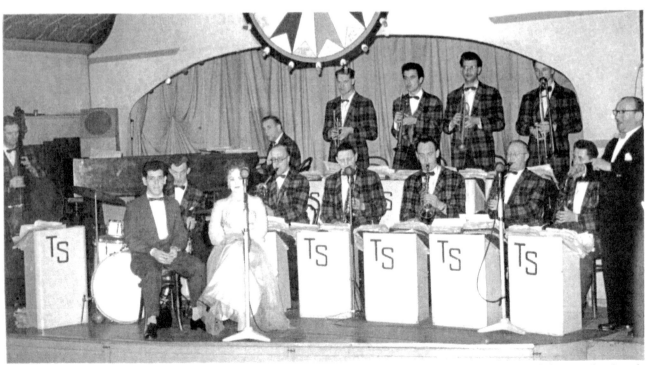

The Tommy Smith Band at the Savoy Ballroom, Oldham, with Tommy on the extreme right. In the band are Ken Henshaw, Ralph Burns and Ray Bickerton (trumpets); Jack Smith (centre of saxes), and Jackie Allan (male vocalist)

the existing band, which included Jimmy Edwards and Bill Garner (saxes), Bert Daniels (bass), Teddy Higham (drums), Bill Heeds (piano) and featured vocalists Lesley Welsh (the 'Blonde Bombshell') and Eddie Mitchell, the Bing Crosby stylist.

The name Bing Crosby reminds me of the biggest mistake I ever made in the music business. In 1951, when I was the bandleader at the same Lido and searching for a good male vocalist, a young hopeful turned up one evening for an audition. He was a dark-haired youth, with a sort of lantern jaw and a good-humoured, lop-sided grin. It appeared that he

was ex-Merchant Navy and had travelled from Liverpool to see me. He had a bundle of musical arrangements under his arm - unusual in those days.

When he sang he sounded so much like Bing Crosby that I thought it was the great man himself at the microphone. He was so good that the musicians applauded him for more, which was even more unusual. However, that was the day of the more aggressive type of singers like Frankie Laine and Johnnie Ray and I told Mike that although I was a great admirer of Crosby and his easy-going style, that wasn't quite what audiences were looking for just then.

Mike Holliday went on to be one of the most sought-after singers in London, recording and broadcasting freely!

The Astoria Ballroom in Plymouth Grove was a very popular venue, featuring a very good band fronted by Tony Stewart. The Chorlton Palais-de-Danse was also popular with the dancers of Manchester and the Bill Webb Band was noted for its star personnel and modern dance band arrangements.

In Bury, the Palais featured music provided by the Jack Cannon Band. This band reigned there for so many years that it seemed it would be there for all time, but nothing goes on forever and inevitably the day came for Jack's departure. When he was eventually replaced it was said he wouldn't have taken the job in the first place, had he known that it wasn't going to be regular! Some local comic labelled the event 'Cannon gets fired'.

The Broadway in Eccles was noted for its cinema downstairs and its popular ballroom above. Many dancers will recall happy times at the Alhambra Palais with the Doug Schofield Band, and the Levenshulme Palais was privileged to retain the services of the Bill Edge Band for many years. The Ashton Palais featured the long engagement of the Raymond Woodhead Band, while another fixture was the Tommy Smith Band at the Savoy Ballroom in Oldham. Tommy had many notable musicians in his line-up, such as Amos Smith, Tommy Hilton, Ralph Burns, Roger Fleetwood, Laurie Holloway and Ronnie Hazelhurst.

North Manchester was well served by the Devonshire Ballroom on Devonshire Street, Broughton (Dyson's); the aforementioned Finnigan's in Queens Road, the Cheetham

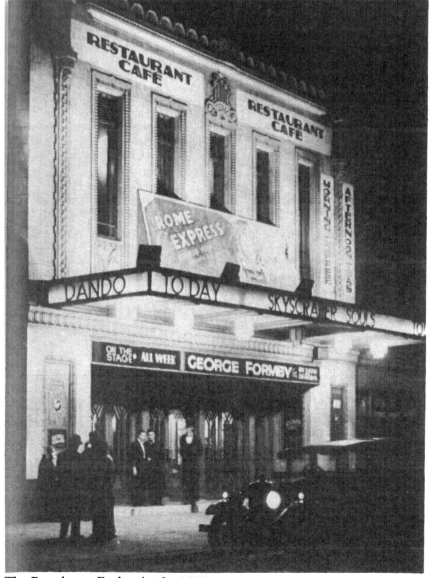

The Broadway, Eccles, in the 1930s

Assembly Rooms and the Higher Broughton Assembly Rooms, to name a few.

My very first paid gig was at the Higher Broughton Assembly Rooms in 1937. The occasion was a wedding and when I first saw the bandleader, Sam Sanderson, I thought he was the bridegroom. He was dressed in immaculate white tie and tails, complete with tall, glossy silk hat, which he wore throughout the evening's dance.

When the bride and the real groom took to the floor in the Bridal Waltz, Sam stepped off the stage and danced around the happy couple, playing 'One Night of Love' on his violin. It was a nice piece of theatre from one of those sentimental gentlemen of that era.

I didn't know until the end of the evening that we had two audiences. It was summer, the ballroom windows were open and my mother and father had been standing outside, patiently waiting to hear my second-hand trumpet sounding off.

During my own dancing years, prior to turning pro musician, I

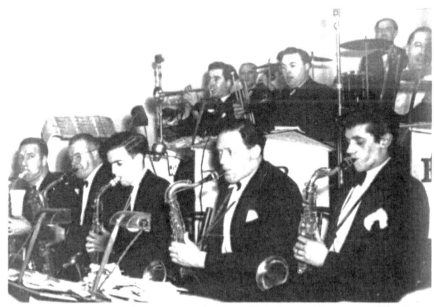

The Bill Edge Band at Levenshulme Palais de Danse, with Ray Bickerton and Harry Pook (trumpets); Freddie Marples and Jack Cosgrove (second and fourth from left) in the saxes

was a regular patron at Dyson's on Devonshire Street each Tuesday - admission 7d. Like most ballrooms of that era, Dyson's relied on dance competitions to attract the crowds. The place was hardly elaborate, but it enjoyed the patronage of good ballroom dancers such as Joe Stewart and his wife Nellie McCauley, Sticker Elliot and Ella Wiseman, and Tango Maishe,

who was noted for his version of the Tango, as the name implied.

One Tuesday my friend Maurice (Chatz) Kelson won the foxtrot contest with his regular partner, Betty Pattison, much to the annoyance of the supporters of a rival contestant. The prize was a set of fireside accessories (it was the day of the coal fire) - tongs, poker, brush and pan, etc - all wrapped up in the pages of the News of the World. We decided it would be wise to leave early so, with the prize under Maurice's arm, we set off, followed by the opposing gang of youths. They broke into a run when we did. I was beginning to wonder what they would do to my features, when there was a nerve-shattering clatter as the fireside set slid from under my friend's arm and crashed to the pavement. It saved our bacon, as the pursuers decided to pick up the pieces and give up the chase.

Each Wednesday we would go to Finnigan's Dance Academy, which was slightly upmarket from Dyson's, with an admission charge of 9d. The academy was then under the

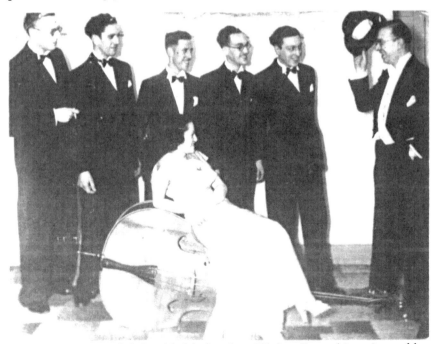

Sam Sanderson (right) with his band at Higher Broughton Assembly Rooms in 1937. Phil Moss is on the right, next to Sam

supervision of Mrs Ryder and Mrs Kerrigan, daughters of founder Jimmy Finnigan. The dancers mentioned above also visited Finnigan's, along with Nat Basso (the boxing promoter) and brother Maurice, the Kersh boys, the three Fraser brothers, the Edelson family and others too numerous to mention.

There were so many venues for ballroom dancers in the same period that I feel a bit shipwrecked in trying to list them all. We had Wantling's of Stanley Grove, Longsight, the 'R.B' at Moss Side, the Gransmoor in Openshaw, the well-known Jimmy Winters Dance Academy, the Downing Street Co-op Hall in Ardwick, Cadman's in Sale - the list goes on and no slight is intended on those I have omitted to mention.

Cadman's was established in 1903 and is Manchester's second oldest dance school after Finnigan's. The school was then in King Street, Stretford, and Mr Cadman ran it with his daughter, Peggy, doing most of the teaching downstairs and

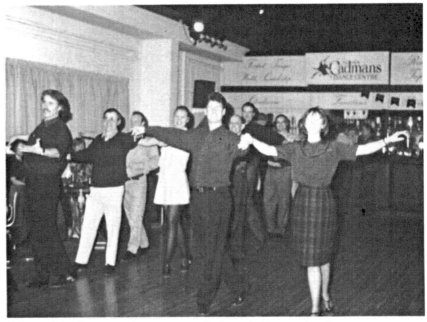

Wayne Newhouse and partner at Cadman's Dance Academy

holding dances in the upstairs ballroom. Vic Ladkin, the next owner, moved the school to Ashfield Road, Sale, when the King Street building had to be demolished; Betty and Geoffrey Morris took over in the sixties, teaching modern ballroom and Latin American.

Cadman's was bought by Wayne Newhouse in 1991 and today it is a very successful dance centre, offering the

experience and enjoyment of dance from children's classes to tea dances.

Ballrooms varied in size and nature, but in those halcyon days they had one thing in common. That very important ingredient was the etiquette - the social graces - of the modern ballroom...

The Etiquette of the Ballroom

The etiquette of ballroom dancing was based on the right of a gentleman to approach a lady for a dance. She was not obliged to accept his invitation, but having refused him, was not expected to take up another offer during the duration of that dance.

It was always a tricky moment. She didn't always know whether the gentlemen could in fact dance and he may have had the same reservation about her. Or how tall would she be when she stood to her full height? Mistakes were common and it wasn't at all unusual to see a short man attempting to steer a taller lady around a crowded floor, with nothing to help him apart from a red face full of cleavage!

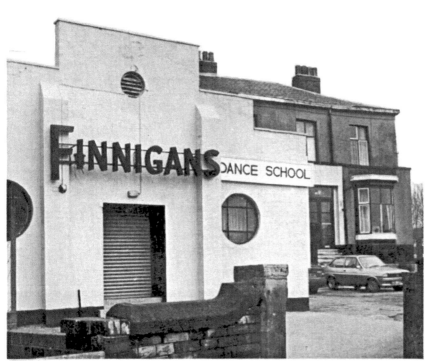

Finnigan's Dance Academy on Queens Road, Cheetham, in 1996

It could sometimes be a bit of a tense situation for a group of girls when a male approached - each not knowing who he had in mind to ask. There was a young lady's feeling of relief when she realised that it was not, in fact, herself that the gentleman had in mind, but with the perverseness we allow ladies, there was also the feeling of being overlooked!

It was the custom at the end of the dance for the gentleman to escort the lady back to the same spot where he had found

her. Another custom was for all dancers to acknowledge the efforts of the orchestra with a brief polite handclap at the end of each dance. Smoking or drinking on the dance floor was strictly taboo and couples were expected to conform to the accepted pattern of each particular dance, thus avoiding collisions on the floor.

In the very early days of ballroom dancing it was usual to have the services of a Master of Ceremonies, who would announce the name of each

dance and watch for any irregularities in the graces I have mentioned. In the larger halls, or on more important occasions, he would be dressed in white tie and tails and white gloves to distinguish him from the rest of the crowd. The whole package didn't prevent dancers from enjoying themselves and it encouraged a standard of behaviour and good manners for the benefit of all.

Sartorial elegance and ballroom decorum went hand-in-glove during those decades of ballroom dancing in Manchester. The ladies invariably wore stylish dresses and no male was allowed to enter the ballroom unless he was wearing a collar and tie. Even when the casual look edged its way on to the scene, there were managements which still insisted on the wearing of the formal necktie and they even went to the length of loaning them out for the evening, free of charge! Dinner dances would see the gentlemen in tuxedos and ladies in elegant evening gowns and it was then commonplace for people to have at least one article in their wardrobe for such occasions.

The bands played their part in all this, dressing in smart band uniforms and all-in-all there would be a feeling of general well-being and pride in the proceedings.

The dancing crowd was made up of many factions. For example, there were the social dancers, happy just to negotiate the floor at their leisure; the keen dancers, darting in and out of the available open spaces to demonstrate their skills; the couples who sat at tables, and the unattached who roamed at will, predators of both sexes.

They say that beauty is in the eye of the beholder, and nowhere is that more true than in the world of ballroom

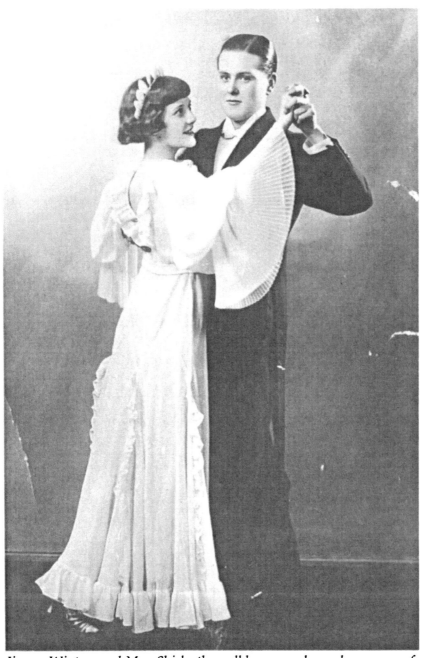

Jimmy Winters and May Shiels, the well known and popular owners of the Jimmy Winters Dance Academy

dancing and dancers. The knockers have described accomplished dancers as 'penguins' and 'prima donnas' and worse; on the other hand, fans and admirers have applauded their poise, elegance and sheer dedication.

But even social dancers complained about how much floor space was taken up by the professionals and semi-pros flashing round the floor. It is a fact that if you had twenty experienced couples sweeping round the average-sized ballroom, it was overcrowded. On the other hand, five times that number of social dancers could be accommodated in the same amount of space.

In the early days of ballrooms, good dancers were courted by managements who relied on dance contests and exhibitions to attract the crowds. 'Jivers', who also needed plenty of space for their gymnastics, were given the cold shoulder and 'No Jiving' notices were prominently displayed in most venues.

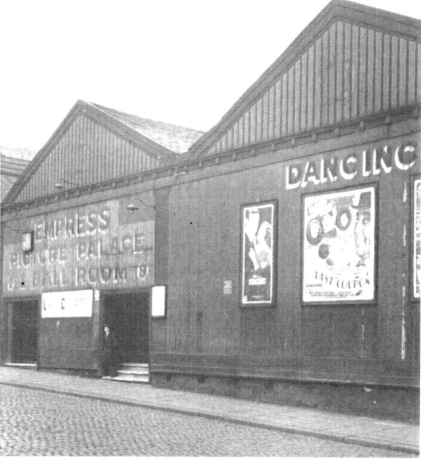

The Empress Picture Palace and Ballroom on Church Street, Pendleton, in the 1930s. The 'Emp' was one of the most popular of the Manchester and Salford ballrooms and attracted thousands of ballroom dancers over a period of many years

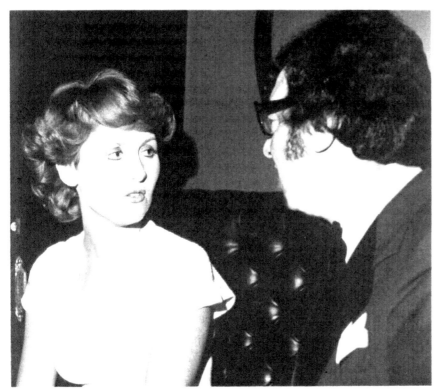

After the pop revolution - Phil Moss with Lulu at the Cat's Whiskers, Oldham

However, when the number of potential jivers began to multiply, the management saw the way things were going and bandleaders began to announce permission for jiving in certain dances. The jivers now had their foot firmly in the door and in the fifties the Jive was recognised as one of the competition dances in the Latin American section.

Then came the sixties, the emergence of the pop scene, and the whole revolutionary exercise was repeated. The popsters took precedence over the jivers, and they needed less space on the floor, doing their own thing, twisting and shaking more or less on the same spot. This was a dream come true for promoters, who could now accommodate huge crowds in a comparatively limited space!

'It happened in Harpurhey a long time ago'

The Harpurhey Baths Ballroom was the scene of the first radio broadcast with my own band, giving it a special place in my memory. So much so, that I recently went to take a picture of the place - Harpurhey revisited. The photo developed, I stared at it over and over again. How well I remembered those steps! There were some half-dozen of them leading up to the doorway, worn by the feet of countless swimmers and dancers over many years.

I had good cause to remember them. My mind went back to the time we held a Wild West Night, with the musicians in cowboy outfits, riding round the ballroom on hired donkeys. But when we planned the event we didn't allow for the poor animals refusing to walk up those steps! It was only when we borrowed planks of wood to give them a surface to walk on that we managed to coax the donkeys into the ballroom so that the Wild West Show could get under way!

They were the same steps negotiated by the singing star Frankie Vaughan, when he sang with us in the early days of his career. I met him quite recently and was surprised that he remembered the place so well.

They were the same steps climbed by Mecca's big shot, Eric Morley, then the managing director of the largest ballroom organisation in the world. He had left his sumptuous offices in London, travelled the two hundred miles to the Rainy City and tracked down the obscure Harpurhey Baths, where he took a seat among a crowd of Palais dancers to see and assess the then little-known Phil Moss Band and Singers. I wasn't kidding myself he had travelled so far to admire the colour of my eyes. As a director

of hundreds of establishments, he had come to see for himself just what was bringing in so many people every night of the week. What he saw was a well drilled and organised outfit, obviously out of its true environment, playing in a North Manchester swimming pool covered by a false floor.

If Eric Morley reads this book he may recall offering me a job at the end of the evening, which I turned down with the appropriate gratitude. Having recently finished many years of touring, I had no wish to jump back on the bandwagon so soon. This was 1952, and it wasn't until 1954, after again being propositioned by Mecca, that I finally accepted a job at the Ritz Ballroom in Manchester. I stayed there for seventeen years and was with the firm, on and off, for twenty-three years in all.

Those very same steps at Harpurhey Baths greeted Fred Barwell, Managing Director of

the Palace and Derby Castle Company in Douglas, Isle of Man. It was Mr Barwell's proud boast that nobody had ever spotted his presence when he secretly came to audition them, so it was sheer luck on my part to see him dodge into the back of the hall one evening. He was almost bent double and took a seat right at the very back. I put my band through all its party tricks until, surprise, surprise, he made himself known and made an offer for the summer season, which I accepted promptly with thanks.

That was the start of a very long career in the Isle of Man - eleven summer seasons in all - at the Derby Castle and the Palace Ballroom and Theatre, and finally at the famous Villa Marina, which had been my long-term target throughout.

I took another long look at those dusty steps at Harpurhey Baths, my stairway to a long and happy association!

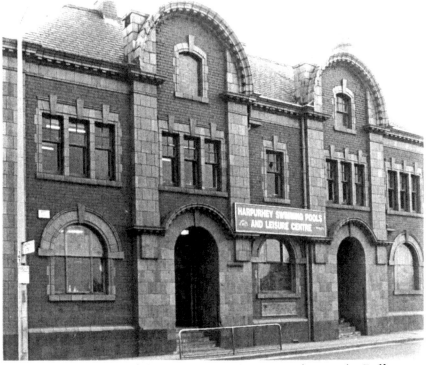

A recent photograph of the entrance to the Harpurhey Baths Ballroom, Rochdale Road. The bands of Ray Allan, Percy Pease and Phil Moss were among the many that appeared there

The Birth of a Band

I was asked recently, 'How long does it take to become a bandleader?'

Well, it can take five minutes or five years and you can't hold a band together unless you have regular work to offer them. The big trick is to find an engagement first and then the musicians follow naturally.

After an absence from my home town of twelve years, many of them playing with the Joe Loss Band, I had an impressive record as a musician, but no experience as a bandleader. But I managed to persuade my old bandleader Percy Pease, who had gone into management, that I could do the job successfully and he gave me my first bandleading job at the High Street Baths Ballroom. Having secured the job first, I had no trouble finding musicians.

The High Street Baths Ballroom

I formed a twelve-piece band and our first engagement was for seven months only at the High Street Baths, starting in September 1950. It was an unknown band which had to prove itself in a short space of time. With the help of the Manchester Evening News, I invited the population of Manchester to choose a name for my band. I knew for sure it was going to be the 'Phil Moss Band', but the newspaper competition went a long way towards making my name known swiftly. Funnily enough, nine suggestions out of ten were for 'Phil Moss and the Rolling Stones'. The Stones had yet to emerge and my band and I were amused at the corny idea - which shows just how wrong one can be!

On our opening night we had a Moss convention, allowing everyone called Moss to get in free of charge - another name-building ploy. But of all the gimmicks I used, and there were many, the illuminated band trick was the ace in the pack. I had all the music stands, uniforms and instruments treated with luminous paint. It didn't show until the house lights went out and the ultra-violet lights came on, but then the whole bandstand lit up like a neon sign. As this happened my singing quartet went into 'Dancing in the Dark'. The idea of using luminous paint and ultra-violet lights came from my experiences in the London theatres, where they were combined to great effect, and the gimmick became a talking point in Manchester's dancing circles. It helped to launch my band into its long and successful run.

On the opening night I wore a wax flower in my buttonhole

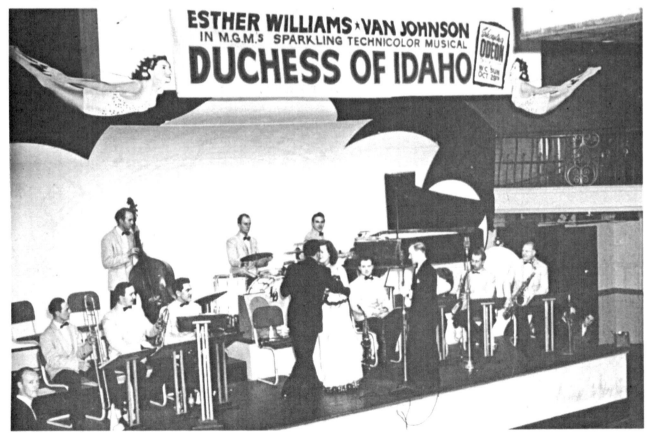

The first Phil Moss Band at the High Street Baths Ballroom in 1950: Bill Limb and Bunny Lewis (trumpets); Russ Stapleford (bass); Billy Brown, Reg Dyson and Jimmy Edwards (saxes); Miff Hill (trombone), and Steve Evans (piano). Vocalist Celia Nicholls is dancing with Phil Moss

but it melted in the heat of the stage lights, much to the guffaws of the musicians, who were noted for their wicked sense of humour. Every evening following I sported a fresh flower, termed 'Phil's Flower', which I presented in turn to the lady with the happiest smile, the most colourful dress, and so on.

The 'Dancing in the Dark' feature initially lasted ten minutes or so, but as its popularity grew, we extended this to about twenty minutes, during which time couples were afforded the opportunity to show their affection for each other - without an audience. One evening a policewoman in plain clothes came in (at the instigation of a rival ballroom manager, I suspect). She had a taste of this High Street 'hospitality' and there followed a big hoo-ha in the press. We were told that in future we could have a partial black-out, but not a complete one. As the 'Dancing in the Dark' feature was not effective unless the

house lights were turned out, it came to an untimely end.

I wasn't unduly upset. It was near the end of my contract and I had already won my wager with my friend and rival bandleader Maurice Mack, about being able to fill the venue in such a short period of time. The popularity of the place was confirmed to me in a letter I received recently. The writer claimed that he and his girlfriend had paid to enter the ballroom, but were kept in the foyer, listening to the band, until another couple left and so made room for them to get in!

Forty-five years on, I still meet scores of ballroom dancers who talk about 'Dancing in the Dark'!

Have Band, Will Travel

The entertainment industry is regarded as one of glamour, but it does have its share of nightmares. For example, there are the dubious joys of travel.

It is possible for a touring band

on one-night stands to play thirty towns in the space of a month. We would travel by coach, boat or 'plane to reach destinations on time, and if you've ever tried to sleep with your head banging on a coach handrail, you will know what it's like.

Even a short journey can present hazards. Some time ago I booked in a quartet to play at a swish hotel in Cheshire. They travelled in two cars and the one containing the pianist and lead guitarist (the melody providers) went into a snowdrift and never arrived at the hotel.

The other car carried the bass player (bum-bum) and the drummer (bang-bang). They did arrive on time and tried to explain to the hostess that they could not possibly provide dance music because the two melody men were missing. The hostess, a gorgeous lady, was aghast. She demanded to know how she could possibly tell the guests, who were arriving in their Rolls-Royces and Mercedes, that the function was off? And what the hell was she to do with the mountains of food and drink? Not to mention the fact that she was responsible for booking the band and the success of the affair. And they were supposed to be musicians, weren't they? They must get on with the job and do the best they could.

Acting on the time-honoured cliché that 'the show must go on' - although nobody has ever said why - the valiant duo set up and started to perform: 'Bum-ching, bum-ching'. The lady organiser played an heroic part, dancing incessantly and shouting out what a marvellous band it was. It didn't deafen people with the tune. It was the 'new' sound, she claimed - the very latest 'big band' sound.

After some twenty minutes of 'bum-ching', the bass player's

Four of Manchester's leading percussionists - Merton Kaufman, Ken Leyland, Amos Smith and Freddie Taylor - outside Stock & Chapman's musical instrument shop on Oxford Road in 1960

nerves were in shreds. 'I've got an idea,' he called to the drummer. 'I'll go to the back of the hall to see what the band sounds like.' With that, he put down his bass and beetled off, probably to the bar. The hostess was undeterred, flouncing all over the place. 'It's even better,' she trilled. 'It's not even as loud as before.' As a publicist, this lady was a world beater.

'I say,' she called out to the drummer, who had been thrashing everything in sight to cover up the absence of the 'bum' section of the dance orchestra. 'Could you possibly play "Moonlight Serenade"?'

'Madam,' came back the drummer, 'what the hell do you think I'm playing?'

A much more worrying aspect of touring is the high incidence of divorce. I was looking at an old picture of my band recently and was shaken when I realised that at least half of the group were no longer with their partners. But there is no great mystery here, when you

consider the lengthy separations and the opportunities for both parties.

Of course, there are times when you can see too much of your spouse, bringing on a fraying of the nerves. Jack Benny, the famous American entertainer, had the answer to that one. He was married for fifty years to the actress Mary Livingston. The day of their Golden Wedding was celebrated on a television programme. The presenter asked Jack how on earth he had managed to stay married to the same lady for fifty years, which by Hollywood standards represented five hundred years. (It has been noted that most marriages in Las Vegas take place early in the day. This is in case it doesn't work out and the couple can return later to have the deal annulled.)

'Well, it is quite simple really,' replied Jack Benny. 'Every single week of our marriage we enjoyed two romantic candlelit evenings. Mary went every Tuesday, and I never missed a Thursday.'

Manchester's Theatreland

Long before television changed the pattern of our lives, local theatres presented live variety shows. Many of these theatres have disappeared. There was the Queens Park Hippodrome in Turkey Lane, Harpurhey; the Alhambra in Openshaw, the Princes Theatre in Oxford Street (closed in 1940) and the Metropole on Ashton Old Road, Openshaw, which closed in 1938 after a run of forty years. The Ardwick Empire, later named the New Manchester Hippodrome, survived until 1961 and I well remember playing there with the Joe Loss Band.

The old Manchester Hippodrome in Oxford Street had a chequered existence, closing down in the thirties to emerge as the Gaumont Cinema. Later the premises became a luxury ballroom with the high-sounding title of Romanoff's. The proprietor was Peter Robinson, a handsome individual with film star looks, an expert wheeler and dealer who knew every gimmick in the book and had everything going for him, except luck. Romanoff's folded and the place was renamed Rotters, but the voodoo persisted and again it was closed, this time for good. Today the site of the once magnificent Gaumont is a piece of waste ground.

Happily I can name at least three survivors which have had their share of adversity but have weathered the storm. The Hulme Hippodrome was taken over by the B.B.C and converted into the B.B.C Playhouse Theatre. It was the home for the broadcasts and concerts of the Northern Dance Orchestra and many other bands, including my own. The theatre closed again in 1986, following the disbanding of the N.D.O, but reopened yet again as the N.I.A centre.

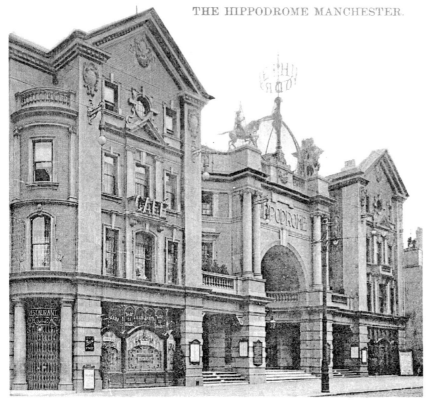

The old Manchester Hippodrome on Oxford Street

The Opera House in Quay Street is an outstanding survivor from the heyday of the theatre. With the popularity of variety on the wane, the Opera House turned to plays and revues, bolstered by the ever-popular pantomime seasons, but gave up the ghost in 1979, much to the horror of Manchester's theatregoers.

To add insult to injury, the building was taken over by Mecca Ltd, with whom I was then employed, and converted into a bingo hall! It was my personal opinion that the Opera House would never make it as a bingo hall and it didn't. After a turbulent period with the powers that be, it reopened as a theatre in 1984. The opening show was 'Barnum', featuring Michael Crawford. My wife and I were at the opening, the show was an outstanding success and the Opera House regained its former glory.

The biggest rival to the Opera House was always the Palace Theatre in Oxford Street. I have always had a soft spot for the Palace, it having been the scene of my audition for the Joe Loss Band in 1946, following my demob from the Royal Air Force. The theatre had a run of well over eighty years, then in 1978, with a shortage of top-line acts and after a tough battle against television and night clubs, it closed.

However, like the Opera House, the Palace rose again from the ashes of theatreland and reopened in 1981. Both theatres continue to present wholesome and exciting shows to the population of Greater Manchester.

The Spice of Life

Theatrical presentations of today owe much to the influence of Andrew Lloyd-Webber and we see two-hour shows such as 'Phantom of the Opera', 'Cats' and 'Me and My Girl', with variety having died a natural death. In the old days a number of variety acts usually occupied the first half of a show, then a top-of-the-bill act, such as a famous band or singer, took the whole of the second half. During the years I toured the theatres of Britain with the Joe Loss band I saw a wide range of supporting acts. There were ventriloquists, tap dancers, fire eaters, sword swallowers, magicians, trapeze artists, jugglers, mind reading acts and hypnotists.

Dancing also had a rôle in the theatres on occasion. Apart from the colourful Adagio dancers, there were exhibitions of Latin American dancing, with the accent on eye-catching dress and steps more in line with cabaret style. In turn, large organisations like Mecca Dancing employed stage acts as cabaret in their ballrooms. This was pre-war, when I was a member of the Doug Swallow Band in 1938, and each Monday morning we had a band call and rehearsal to accompany the acts, who were contracted for one week.

In addition to the stand-up comedians, singers of all descriptions, multi-instrumentalists, strong men and escapologists, there were the animals. Most of these came to the stage via the circus and they included dog acts and performing sealions, who would do amazing balancing tricks, then join in the applause by clapping their flippers. There were the pony acts with their trick riders and the ponies tapping the floor with their

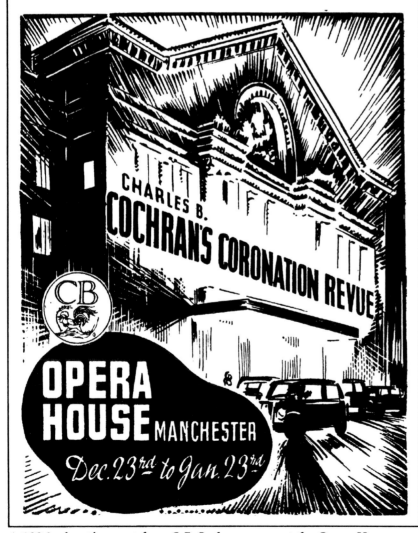

A 1936 advertisement for a C B Cochran revue at the Opera House

hooves in answer to the trainer's questions. One of the more original acts I recall was a hurdle race round the stage, with greyhounds ridden by monkeys. The monkeys were tied on the dogs' backs and dressed in gaudily coloured jockey outfits.

The professional strong men lifted huge weights with their poundage prominently displayed on them. There were the usual comics in the audience, claiming the weights were faked, but these were always silenced by an invitation from the stage for the barrackers to join in the lifts, with a cash prize for the winner. Escapologists were trussed up in chains and bolts and had to escape within a time limit.

A popular act was 'Datas', the memory man, who could tell you the result of any sporting event over the last century.

When asked by a member of the audience for the winner of the Football Association Cup in say, 1912, he would stagger the questioner by giving the correct answer, plus the names of the players in both teams, the name of the referee and the attendance figures for good measure! It was said the only time that Datas slipped up was when he was asked for the winner of an event which had taken place only two days before.

Mind reading acts were always in demand, with one of the performing duo sitting on the stage blindfolded whilst his assistant moved amongst the audience, picking up objects such as rings and watches. The assistant would ask the mindreader to describe the object and the description was always correct, thanks to some prearranged code between the two of them.

'Claude' was an amusing magician who started his act by writing the word 'Claude' on a board and easel. He changed this to 'Great Claude' when he received the applause for his first trick and after more successful tricks it became 'Mighty Claude' and eventually 'Claude Almighty'. On making a hash of the next trick he would look shamefaced and alter his status back to 'Claude'.

There was a hilarious incident at the Palace Theatre in Oxford Street when 'Katinka', the renowned hypnotist, was appearing for the week. Her act was to hypnotise giant snakes, which coiled around her body to the accompaniment of 'Snake Charmer', played by the pit orchestra, conducted by Charlie Windsor. She provided a spectacular finale to her act by bringing on a giant crocodile from the side of the stage and then proceeding to hypnotise it. When the reptile was under the influence it was lifted on to two chairs in the classic levitation position, with its entire length as stiff as a board, and two members of the audience were invited to come up and sit on it.

There are various stories about what happened next on that particular evening. Some say the spotlights were too bright for the poor croc; others maintain that the reptile came out of the 'fluence prematurely. The fact is, its body went limp suddenly and gave way, unseating the two daring riders, who fell into the middle of the pit orchestra, followed by the crocodile. Musicians are not particularly noted for their bravery and the scatter for cover brought the music of 'Snake Charmer' to a dramatic halt. The crocodile was eventually re-harnessed and led away.

That is just another reason for not putting your daughter on the stage, Mrs Worthington!

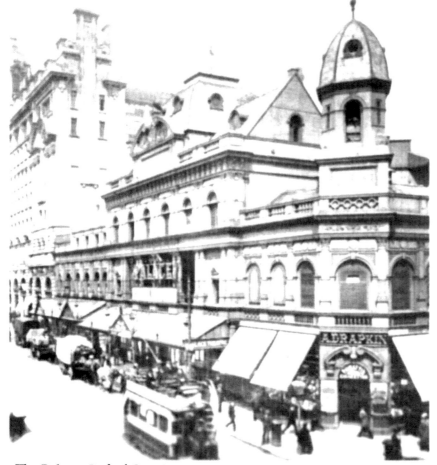

The Palace, Oxford Street

The Rise and Fall of the Big Band Era

Many theories have been advanced to explain the rise in popularity of the 'big bands' and then their disappearance into obscurity in later years. I can assure you that none of the big-name bands found fame overnight, and each one could tell a story of the struggle for recognition in times of adversity. This, of course, applied to bands from the provinces, London and America in equal measure.

Before the arrival of television, radio relied heavily on bands, and in turn radio was the quickest route to public acclaim for the big bands. Jack Payne's was the first resident band to be appointed by the B.B.C in 1928 and his signature tune, 'Say it with Music', made him a household favourite with millions of listeners. He was succeeded later by Henry Hall. ('This is Henry Hall speaking.')

Each evening the B.B.C had a two-hour band feature. Every Saturday we would hear Ambrose and his band, with singers Sam Browne, Elsie Carlisle, Anne Shelton and others. The Friday night slot belonged to Harry Roy (the original 'Hotcha-ma-Chotcha'), featuring the Tiger Ragamuffins, Ivor Moreton and Dave Kaye. Tuesday was taken up by Lew Stone, with Al Bowlly and Nat Gonella. The other evenings were shared by bands like Geraldo, Sidney Lipton, Roy Fox, Billy Ternent, Maurice Winnick and many others.

During my many years of broadcasting with the Joe Loss Band, the announcer would often invite listeners to roll up the carpet and dance to their favourite band without charge. Television latched on to this idea years later, when Victor Sylvester presented his weekly 'Dancing Club' programme. There was a section where dance instruction was given in detail, with the same invitation to 'roll up the carpet' and join in.

Radio was very kind to the big bands, but when television took over, with its endless parade of films, plays, quiz and game shows and soap operas, the spectacle of a large number of musicians sitting reading music looked very old hat indeed. A new generation was now watching music, with all its antics, instead of listening, and so the advent of television had to be one of the factors behind the free fall of the big bands.

Television made an impact in another way, too. There was no longer any need to brave the elements in order to be entertained. So the big venues, the ballrooms and theatres which had employed large bands, were also disappearing. Some bandleaders were quick to heed the red light. Jack Jackson, noted West End bandleader, turned to being a disc jockey - probably the most entertaining of them all. Maurice Winnick, the Manchester bandleader who enjoyed a fairytale success in London, turned to promoting television game shows such as 'What's My Line' and 'Twenty Questions'.

The B.B.C, which had provided so many opportunities for musicians, was now courting a

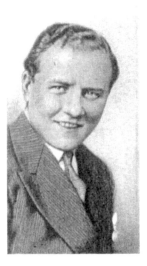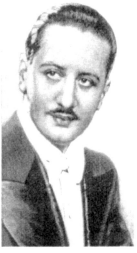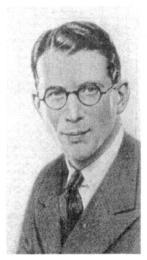
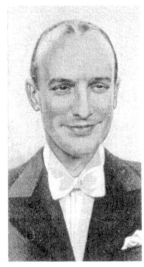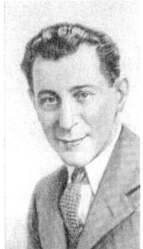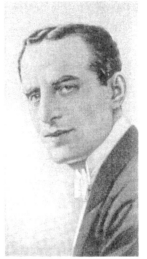

Bandleaders on the B.B.C. Top: Jack Payne, Geraldo, Henry Hall. Bottom: Roy Fox, Lew Stone, Ambrose

whole flock of disc jockeys to take their place. The big bands had become dispensable and being vulnerable, they were fighting for their very existence. I know of one now very famous disc jockey who left his bar serving duties to stand in for a resident D.J who had failed to turn in that evening. He went on to become a very highly paid radio personality just like that. On the other hand, he could have spent a lifetime studying music, to finish up crying into the bell of his saxophone like so many others.

The first time I ever saw records being played in the ballroom was when I had a season at the Rex Ballroom in Stockport in 1951. The manager had the bright idea of inviting dancers to bring in their own favourite dance records and these would be played in place of the interval each evening. The idea caught on to such an extent that ballrooms extended the time allocated. Then somebody was employed as a disc jockey as a

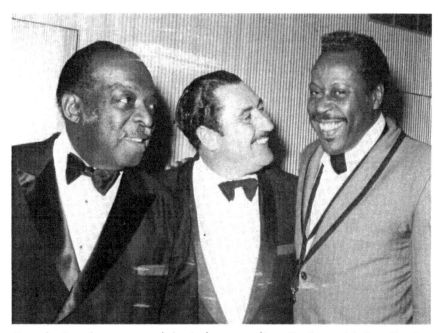

Ronnie Caryl, trumpeter/pianist/arranger/bandleader, with bandleader Count Basie and saxophonist Eddie 'Lockjaw' Davis

fixture and there was no longer a need to engage a second band. Live music was on the slippery slope!

The collapse of live music had ominous side effects. Sales of musical orchestrations by famous publishers dried up and

their wares were left to gather dust on the shelves. Musical instrument dealers were also fighting a losing battle in trying to sell their instruments to an ever decreasing army of players. At one time there were six of them in Oxford Road, Manchester, and all were

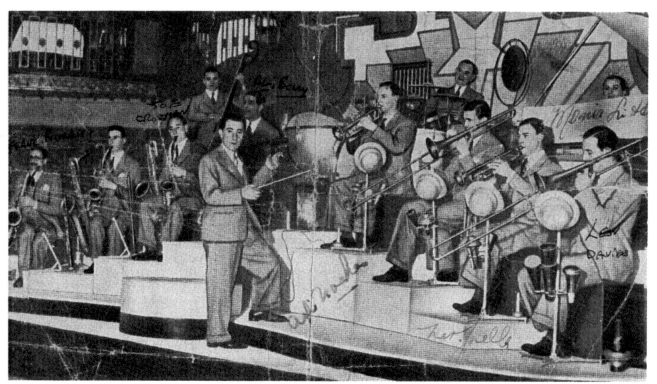

The Lew Stone Band at the Ritz in Manchester in the 1930s. On the photograph are Lew Stone, Al Bowlly (guitar, vocals), Nat Gonella (trumpet), Alfie Noakes (trumpet), Joe Crossman (alto sax), Tiny Winters (bass), Bill Harty (drums), Monia Litter (piano), Lew Davies (trombone), Harry Berly (sax) and Joe Ferrie (trombone)

thriving. Today there is one survivor from that era, the Johnny Roadhouse musical instrument shop.

Perhaps the main reason for the demise of the big band sound was the appearance on the scene of the 'groups' in the early sixties. There must be changes in all walks of life and so it was with the music business. Pop music was new, easy to understand and suited the new ways of dancing of the rising generation. On the other hand, big band music was progressing to such technical heights that the fun-loving adolescents of the post-war baby boom found it difficult to digest, whereas they took the modern, simple, repetitive patterns in their stride. It would take a separate book to expound on this transformation of the musical scene, and to do so would give me much pain and make me few friends!

Coinciding with the problem of the 'vanishing' big bands in the towns and cities of England, there was a similar situation in the U.S.A. Famous bands were being cut down in size and some disappeared altogether. Rather than reduce their status, some of the really large bands embarked on world tours, among them the renowned Woody Herman (and his Herd) and the outstanding Stan Kenton and his Dance Orchestra.

I was lucky enough to play opposite both these bands: with Stan Kenton at the Burtonwood U.S.A.F. Base and Woody Herman at Blighty's Dance Club in Farnworth. The two stars were both very dedicated to their profession and continued to tour world-

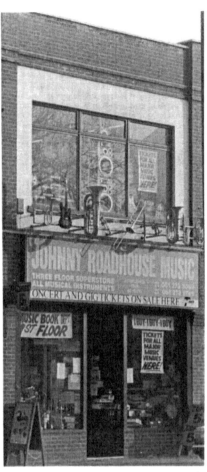

The Johnny Roadhouse Music Shop on Oxford Road in 1996

wide until ill health overtook them.

Another American 'glamour band' that managed to avoid the general demise was that of the trumpet virtuoso Harry James. The band was featured in many big musical films, which helped Harry to stave off the evil day, so to speak. Then he, too, took to the road on tour.

When the professional bands were shunted into the sidelines, some still fought on, through optimism, self-belief or just plain love of the business. One of these was led by a man who at twenty was the youngest 'name' leader, and the oldest when he died in his eighties. He managed to keep a large band fully employed for all of those sixty years and for that reason alone he deserves a king-size roll on the drums. I refer, of course, to the late, great Joe Loss.

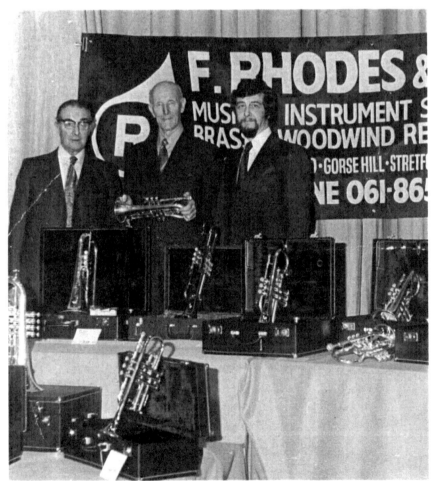

Musical instrument dealer Fred Rhodes (left) and his son Granville (right) with Jack Macintosh, famous recording trumpet and cornet soloist

Mr Joe Loss - Showman Extraordinaire

The Joe Loss Band was considered to be the best large band for ballroom dancing in the country and playing for ballroom dancing was Joe's first and last love in all the activities of his band. He was featured in all the major dance competitions, at home and abroad, appeared for many long years on 'Come Dancing' and received the Carl-Alan Award for services to the ballroom industry on several occasions.

Most of Joe's bandleading contemporaries had show bands, hotel bands, powerhouse units or comedy bands, but Joe was at his best going out and about amongst the Great British Dancing Public. He appeared regularly at all the biggest venues and at most of the important occasions, and he was also the adopted darling of the provincial cities, in particular our own city of Manchester.

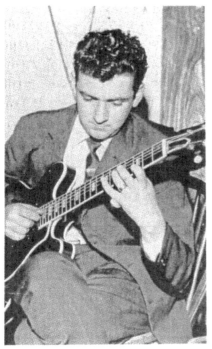

Ace guitarist Bob Gill joined the Phil Moss Band at the Ritz and afterwards featured in the bands of Joe Loss, Ken Mackintosh and Victor Sylvester

Although the band was London-based, Joe always employed several provincial players and among the Manchester contingent were trombonists Harry Symons and Ken Wray, trumpeters Sid Pollitt, Billy Burton and myself; saxophonists Arthur Lester and Alan Wood, drummer Dave King and guitarist Bob Gill.

I shan't dwell on the details of Joe's career, which is well documented already, but on the man behind the baton, which he wielded with the magic of a genuine showman. He gave so many opportunities to individual musicians, including myself. After six years in the R.A.F I returned to Manchester in a very ill-fitting demob suit, wondering how to pick up the threads of Civvy Street again. Joe's band was appearing at the Palace Theatre, I asked him for an audition in the band, which he granted and he followed that by giving me a fresh start in life.

Long before television ruled all, Joe realised that people were watching music in preference to listening to it and so he made visual entertainment his priority. We hear today of charisma, panache and other qualities; Joe had them all in abundance and as a showman he had no peers. He was a dapper individual, always immaculately dressed and with an hypnotic smile on his aquiline features. He gyrated in front of his band with the grace of a ballroom dancer, selling his band and himself with an expertise that many leaders of industry would do well to follow.

He was about 5ft 7in in height but he had the habit of holding his hand high when he shook hands, at the same time raising on his toes to complete the

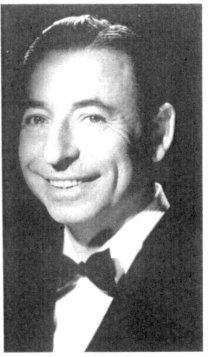

illusion. When you looked into those fine mesmeric eyes you saw a man in complete control of himself and those around him.

He gave himself the star treatment - five star - and was aware of the pitfalls of familiarity and the advantages of mystique, so it was possible to work in his band and yet rarely speak to him. Talking, of course, was taboo on stage and when sessions finished he was whisked off to his private dressing room, where he would have a complete change of clothes. He re-emerged refreshed and raring to go for the next session, his long black hair glistening after a good 'friction' and you could almost hear the starch crackling in his crisp, snow-white laundry.

Joe always played hard to get. If you telephoned his office to offer the most prestigious engagement, a voice would promise to 'let you know very soon'. Even the Queen (we were regular visitors to the Palace) seemed in awe of him when he conducted the National Anthem in a fashion that would have put Laurence Olivier to shame.

The last day of the Villa Marina season on the Isle of Man was always marked with a party given for the entertainers, management, staff and civic dignitaries. Speeches were made by the Mayor, Town Clerk and Borough Treasurer - each in nervous 'let's get it over' style - to which hardly anyone listened.

I was having a few drinks at the bar when I noticed that the hubbub was dying down and 'shush, shush' sounds were coming from both ends of the room. These were being made by Joe Loss's manager and secretary to ensure that the last speaker - the Great Man himself - would be heard in complete silence. It wasn't until you could hear a pin drop that Joe would deliver his unhurried, carefully measured vote of thanks to the entire gathering. It was an object lesson in commanding total submission from an audience - pure, vintage Joe Loss!

In order to avoid autograph hunters, Joe spent leisure moments signing hundreds of small photographs and every member of the band carried

some of these around to dish out as requested.

On the night I finally left the band (at the Winter Gardens, Blackpool, in 1950) Joe's manager informed me that the great man wished to speak to me at the end of the evening. When I entered his room, still wearing my band jacket, he motioned for me to sit down while he paced up and down, Hollywood style. 'Phil,' he said dramatically (Joe was always dramatic), 'you have been with me all these years, always punctual, sober, well groomed and professional in every way and I can't let you leave without some token of my esteem.'

I sat quite still as he paused for effect. I was now convinced it wasn't just a gold watch. Maybe a gold clock?

'Phil,' he commanded, 'pass me one of those photographs.' He pointed to a stack of them on his desk. He signed it with a flourish and I transferred it to my pocket with about twenty similar ones. He inclined his head sadly and that was the finale. I left the room in a

silence you could cut with a knife, closing the door as if it were made of egg shells.

He wasn't without humour and if members of the band were larking about on coach journeys he would tell us to behave - or he would play his violin! This threat allegedly originated after an incident one night at the Liverpool Empire. Joe used to play a short solo on his violin, without bothering to tune up for the small item, until one night one of the comics in the band let down his strings. This had catastrophic results and it was apparently the last time he ever performed his party piece!

One day I found him listening rapturously to a high-powered U.S.A recording. When I asked him why he didn't allow us to play in that fashion he was genuinely shocked. 'Phil,' he said, 'this is my pleasure. The other is my business.'

The Joe Loss Band and my own shared the honours at the Prince Charles Ball at the Piccadilly Plaza Hotel in Manchester, which had all the local big-wigs in attendance. When Joe's large band finished its session there was the usual standing ovation and it looked as if it would be a case of following the Lord Mayor's Show for the lesser Phil Moss Band. I snatched up my trumpet and crashed in with the time-honoured tune, 'Charlie is my darling, my darling, my darling', and the crowd loyally took up the chant and clapped their hands. Prince Charles rose from his seat at the top table and acknowledged my gesture with a slight bow, which I promptly returned, and the day was saved for yours truly.

Joe passed me later on the bandstand, murmuring, 'Well, who's a clever boy then?' My look of appreciation could have earned me an Oscar. 'Thanks, Joe,' I said, 'You were a wonderful teacher!'

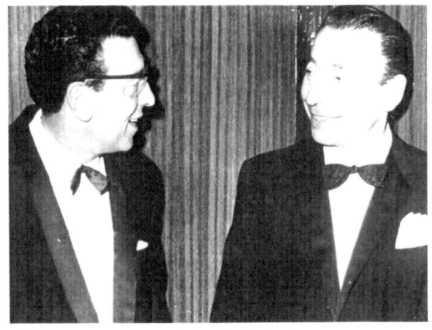

Phil Moss and Joe Loss reunited at the Ritz in 1957

Victor Sylvester

Victor Sylvester's contribution to the ballroom industry was vast, first as a former world champion dancer and later with England's leading strict tempo dance orchestra. He was to dancing what Heinz is to baked beans, yet I can't think of a single musician who wouldn't shudder at the thought of being stranded on a desert isle with nothing to hear but Victor Sylvester's music! Nevertheless, he was probably the most widely-known, successful bandleader in the country and his records sold in their millions all over the world.

His fame started long before his success as a bandleader, when he became the World's Modern Ballroom Dancing Champion in 1922. In that capacity he saw that there wasn't a single big-time band catering exclusively for ballroom dancers and in 1936 he formed his first band for that specific purpose. Simplicity was the keynote of his success and a year later he made his first broadcast. The Victor Sylvester Band went on to make thousands of broadcasts for the B.B.C in the famous 'Request' programme and there were many appearances in the 'Dancing Club' television show. He was awarded the O.B.E in 1962.

Sylvester was a pianist, although he didn't play in his own band, which included Oscar Grasso (violinist), Eddie Macauley and Charlie Pude (pianos), 'Poggy' Pogson (saxes and clarinet), Victor Parker (string bass) and Ben Edwards (drums). The signature tune was, aptly, 'You're Dancing on my Heart'. The music was simple in the extreme, based on simple melodies played in strict tempo as laid down by the Dance Teachers' Association. Four bars introduction from the two pianos, then the melody played by one instrument only at a time - violin or saxophone. There was no section work to hinder the tempo and there were no brass instruments, and when the band was augmented for any reason, it was done with the addition of three more saxes. The music was easy on the ear and it made dancing so much easier. There were no pretensions to entertain and no vocalists, which was the biggest single bone of contention between bands and the dancing public.

I first met Victor Sylvester at the Albert Hall in London, when we were playing for the World Ballroom Championships. Four famous bands were engaged to deal with that dancing marathon, which started at midday and continued until 2.00am the following morning. They were the Joe Loss Band, of which I was then a member, Oscar Rabin, Victor Sylvester and Edmundo Ros, who played for the Latin American events. I found Victor to be a modest gentleman of good humour and laid back personality, with a simple, uncomplicated approach to the ballroom industry. He always looked physically fit and I noticed that he ate and drank sparingly from the refreshments available.

The next time we met was when he visited the Ritz in Manchester and broke all existing records at the box office - the management said that patrons were applying for tickets weeks before his appearance. Considering the existence of so many famous bands, knocking themselves to pieces with high-powered musical arrangements and frenzied showmanship, one could only marvel at the simplistic success of Victor Sylvester. A famous politician would have been prompted to say, 'Never was so much success attained with so little effort.'

That same success earned fabulous sums of money for Britain in the export market, making one wonder why Victor Sylvester never progressed further in the Honours lists.

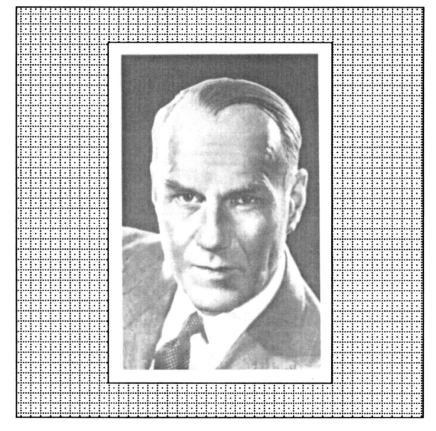

The Mecca Way

Back in the days when ballroom dancing was first becoming the most popular social activity in the country, I remember seeing advertisements such as, 'A Grande Dance will be held at the Downing Street Co-op Hall. Admission 1/- including Refreshments (tea and biscuit). Band in attendance.' Before very long, available halls above Burton's the tailors and Co-op halls had been converted into local ballrooms, with small, semi-pro bands doing the honours. Town halls, assembly rooms and a whole host of small venues jumped on the bandwagon, all combining to make ballroom dancing a real growth industry.

At the same time two gentlemen, Carl L Heimann and Alan B Fairley, were quietly and assiduously building up a chain of large ballrooms in major town centres and this eventually became the biggest chain of dance halls in the world - Mecca Dancing. There were other big fish, of course, like the Rank Organisation, but they were primarily cinema people and never seriously threatened Mecca. Carl Heimann was Mecca's up-front man, with canny Scot Alan Fairley in the background.

When I first joined the company in 1938 as a playing musician Mecca owned just eight halls, including the Ritz in Manchester. In contrast to the local halls which opened one or two nights each week, Mecca coined the slogan, 'Twice a day, the Mecca way', and their ballrooms opened every afternoon and evening six days a week. They were also open on Sunday evenings, when they were run as Sunday clubs for members only. Mecca ballrooms featured not one, but two professional bands, modern décor, cabaret spots and every

refinement possible, so adding a new dimension to public dancing entertainment.

In the 1930s some major ballrooms set aside an area in one corner of the hall, adjacent to the stage, which was christened the 'pen'. It was occupied by a number of professional dancers of both sexes who were there to partner patrons who had purchased tickets at the box office, either singly or in rolls. The tickets were 6d each - 3d going to the company and 3d to the pro dancer - and they were bought by dancers who wished to be sure of a partner during the session.

The system had been used at the Roseland Ballroom in New York and gave birth to that best-selling tune, 'Ten Cents a Dance'. The words went, 'Ten cents a dance, that's what they pay me, that's how they weigh me down,' finishing with the phrase, 'So come on big boy, ten cents a dance.' Well-known Manchester dancer Jack Binks

was in the 'pen' at the Astoria Ballroom, Charing Cross Road, London, before introducing it at the Ritz in Manchester in the thirties, where he became the manager. At the beginning of each afternoon and evening session the occupants of the 'pen' were expected to dance together to create an atmosphere, in a manner known as 'dressing the floor'.

Dancing couples (or courting couples) invariably occupied seats at the tables around the ballroom or those in the balcony café. The 'picking up' area was situated at the back of the hall, where people could mix freely and the gents could invite unescorted ladies to dance without the embarrassment of being observed if they were refused. The standing area was in my opinion a very important ingredient in the box office success of a ballroom and a natural for fostering relationships. The slogan 'We make couples out of singles' was prophetic and many a romance began in the secluded

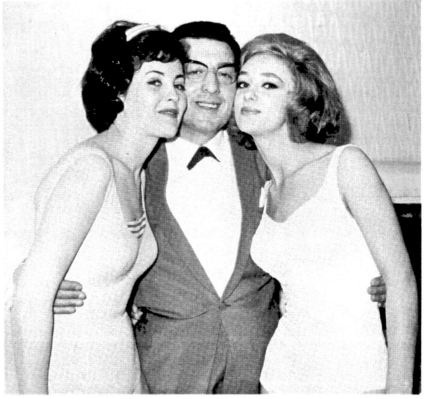

The Miss Wales beauty competition at the Ritz Ballroom in 1956. The winner was Gaynor Cornforth on the right

zone known as the standing area.

The wise manager presented a policy which appealed to as many dancers as possible. Monday could be advertised as 'Popular Night', with a 'Happy Hour' during which drinks prices were reduced. Tuesday was very often 'Good Dancers' Night', when the keen dancers were encouraged to practise and polish up their movements. Wednesday, the mid-week prop, was sometimes announced as 'Novelty Night', with 'Go as you Please' contests and every dance an 'Excuse me' dance. Thursday was often a 'Singles and Unattached' evening - sometimes the 'Lonely Hearts Club'. Friday, always a winner, was usually tagged 'Gala Night' - and 'Free Gift Night', with any free gifts and novelties we could drum up.

Saturday, the big one, was

'Saturday Night Spectacular', in which we threw the book at the crowd, with balloon showers, streamers and blowers and a mixture of every conceivable gimmick to sustain the atmosphere. When City had played United in the afternoon, all the balloons were blue and red and I asked the dancers to keep them in the air as long as they could - the colour of the last balloon determined the 'team of the night'.

Sunday was Club night, to comply with Sunday regulations, when we welcomed all workers in the cinemas, clubs, etc, who had been working themselves on the previous six evenings. It was called 'Continental Night' for many years.

In the constant battle for patronage, many ballrooms offered cheaper admission deals in the shape of season tickets. However, there were

obvious drawbacks to this enterprise for both dancers and managements - the tickets were easily transferable - and the scheme eventually died a natural death.

When a patron entered a Mecca ballroom he or she unwittingly became a statistic. We kept nightly records of attendances, the weather conditions and any counter-attractions that evening. If there was just one patron fewer in the ballroom that night than in the previous year, we were accorded a 'down'. And if we were just one up, it was a very welcome 'up'.

All Mecca ballrooms were listed in a league table with the one recording the most 'ups' going to the top of the list. There was therefore a scramble by bandleaders and managers alike, trying to avoid the bottom of the table and what could be the 'last drop'. There were bonuses for those who did well and brickbats for those in the basement. If Mecca's system wasn't exactly the law of the jungle, it was certainly a recipe for endeavour and survival.

One morning a week at the Ritz there was a meeting in the manager's office for the key figures in management, the catering staff, even the cleaners, and we aired our views, observations and grievances without fear or favour. Ballroom dancing had come of age - from a pleasant recreation to an exact science.

Jack Binks

The manager of the Ritz Ballroom and and director of Mecca Ltd, Jack Binks (known as J.B.), was a man who could inspire you or reduce you to a jelly with equal ease. A week before the start of my much publicised engagement at the Ritz Ballroom, several of my key musicians accepted another job which didn't entail afternoon

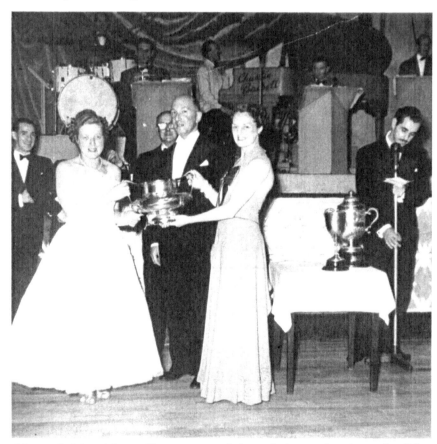

Mr and Mrs Moss Chaytow receiving their rosebowl at the Ritz Ballroom. Frank Gibson is on the left and Ritz manager Jack Binks is on the right. The Charlie Bassett Band at the rear

sessions. I expected a rough passage when I went to Jack's office to tell him what had happened and give him the opportunity to engage another band. Instead, he gazed at me with complete composure, saying he did not know who these men were, nor did he care.

'I didn't engage them,' he said. 'I engaged a man called Phil Moss, and where he is, there will be a good band, and more importantly, a very successful one.' I left Jack's office feeling ten feet tall.

The engagement my original men had accepted folded some time later through poor attendances. During that same period, the cloakrooms at the Ritz had to be doubled in size to accommodate the surge in business!

Jack Binks could be equally forthright in the opposite direction. When the famous Ray Ellington Quartet were engaged to appear with us for two weeks, Danny Segal, the box office manager, and I were detailed to meet them. They arrived on the Monday morning in a vehicle which had a large sign on the back saying, 'You are now following the Ray Ellington Quartet'.

Whilst the band gear was being piled in the foyer I escorted Ray to the band room which I normally shared with the other resident leader, Charlie Bassett. Ray took one look at the room, which admittedly was only slightly larger than a dog kennel, and flatly refused to squeeze his stuff into it, comparing the accommodation to the Black Hole of Calcutta. I offered to move out and share the assistant manager's room during his stay, so he would have the band room to himself, but he remained adamant on the subject. We tramped back to the waiting band and luggage with nothing resolved.

Then Jack Binks arrived. 'Good morning, everybody,' he said. 'Any problems?'

'Yes, sir,' said Danny Segal. 'Mr Ellington finds his accommodation unsuitable.'

Jack managed to look genuinely sorry. I wouldn't have been surprised if he had burst into tears. 'I'm really sorry to hear that,' he said sadly. He waved his well manicured hand in the direction of the huge poster which announced the sensational engagement of the Ray Ellington Quartet. 'Tell me, Mr Ellington,' he continued. 'Are you really staying with us for the next fortnight, or do we have to take this bill down?'

There followed a deafening silence, during which Ray Ellington motioned for his cases to be taken down to the band room, and Jack Binks continued on his leisurely way with as

much fuss as a bishop presiding over a garden party.

Datal Attractions

Every ballroom celebrated the most popular of the seasonal festivities, such as Christmas and New Year, but in order to sustain all-the-year round business we were obliged to exploit every occasion possible, including some which were really out of our province. Even the Chinese New Year was observed, when we invited Chinese students and others to enjoy their celebrations in the Ritz Ballroom. Chinese lanterns were hung everywhere and we even made a long papier mâché dragon for the ritual routine.

To honour Scotland's most famous poet, on Rabbie Burns Night my name was changed to McMoss and there were kilts, Highland Flings, Gay Gordons, Loch Lomond and Annie Laurie

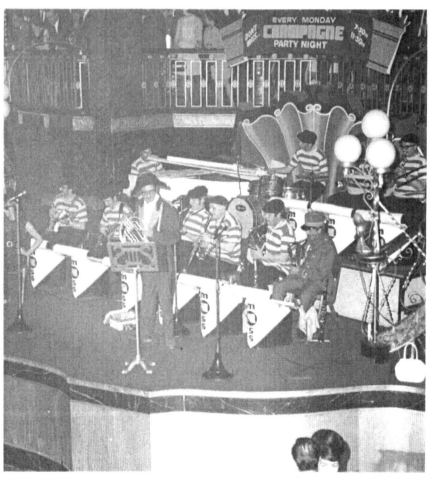

Bastille Night at the Ritz in 1966. The band is attired in typical French clothing, with Phil Moss as Napoleon

thrown in the deep end. We couldn't cope with tossing the caber, but there were tug-of-war contests. It was a night when we all 'belonged to Glasgow'.

St Patrick's Night was always a winner at the box office. We circulated every known Irish and Catholic organisation for miles around and this time the attraction was Phil o'Moss and his Leprechauns. All the balloons released were green, all the musicians and staff wore shamrocks, which were also presented to patrons. 'Irish eyes were smiling' as never before and the Irish jig was something to see, performed to the wildly Gaelic tune of 'The Irish Washerwoman'.

On French Bastille Night my band dressed in berets, striped waistcoats and sunglasses. French national flags decorated the ballroom and I announced all the dances in French (pinched from the dictionary). I was supposed to sound like Maurice Chevalier, but only managed to resemble the voice of the barman in Coronation Street. Romance was the musical theme, with 'J'Attendrai', 'La Vie en Rose', etc, giving way in the end to the colourful 'Can Can'.

Welsh Wales, look you, was never overlooked in our diary for dancers. On St David's Day the Ritz Ballroom became the 'Land of My Fathers' for the evening and we made sure there was 'A Welcome in the Hillside' for all. The day had a special significance for me as I met my wife, Joan, when she was a W.A.A.F. driver at St Davids itself in Pembrokeshire. On V.E. Day I played the 'Last Post' and 'Reveille' to 3,000 airmen in the Cathedral there.

Easter Sunday and Monday were great money-spinners, with miniature eggs for all patrons. A fondly-remembered feature was the Easter Bonnet Parade (ladies wore hats in those elegant days), followed by the Grand Easter Parade itself, with all couples marching arm-in-arm round the ballroom to the famous tune of the same name. It was one of the graces of the ballroom of long ago. It was intriguing that Irving Berlin (of Jewish faith) should write 'Easter Parade' and 'White Christmas', celebrating the two holiest days of the Christian calendar.

Working on the assumption that everyone must have parents, Mother's Day and Father's Day were always anniversaries to be cherished. All mothers and fathers were acknowledged with small gifts, even if they were only pipe-cleaners for the gents and embroidered hankies for the ladies.

St Valentine's Night never failed to attract big attendances and there was a novelty competition for the most original Valentine card. We had the 'kissing arch', which each couple was expected to pass through, with a brief kiss, before moving on to make room for the next couple. On St Valentine's Night this really earned its keep, being used in all the waltzes played. The band dutifully waded through the sweetheart tunes from 'Funny Valentine' to 'I'll Be Your Sweetheart' and towards the evening's end we had a hilarious competition for the funniest proposal of marriage delivered on the stage.

Every Pancake Tuesday we

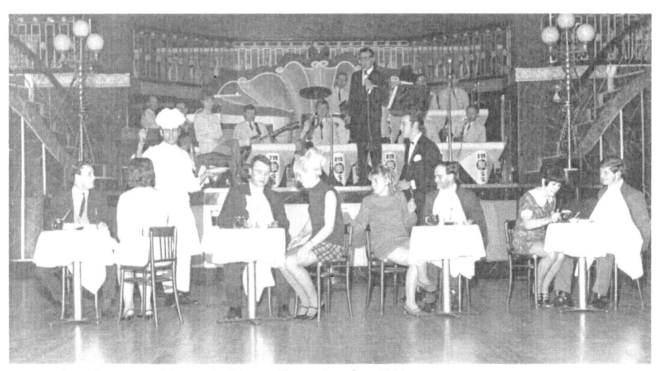

A pancake eating competition at the Ritz on Shrove Tuesday, 1964

featured a 'Tossing the Pancake' competition, followed by the 'Pancake Eating Contest', which was always greeted by roars of raucous laughter. Four couples were seated at different tables, the ladies had to toss up the pancakes (compliments of the chef), then feed them to the gents, who sat with their arms behind their backs. Each had a drink to help them along. The sight of the girls shovelling the gooey mass down the throats of the gents - whose eyes were bulging out - to try and finish the lot first, was only surpassed by the arrival of the prize - another four pancakes!

Perhaps it is in the character of English people to be modest about our past glories, for St George's Day never seemed to rouse as much patriotic fervour as the other national days I have mentioned. Nevertheless, the ballroom was always festooned with Union Jacks (why do some people hang

them upside down?) and we played every conceivable tune associated with the Navy, Army and Royal Air Force. These were usually in the most appropriate tempos of the Military Two-Step and Barn Dances. We worked hard to melt down the reserve of that stiff upper lip and generally managed to convince the dancers that 'There'll Always be an England'!

Halloween Night, with Vampires and 'things that go bump in the night', was another favourite in the dancer's diary. We poor old musicians had to cut large holes in our masks to get the instruments to our mouths. The competitions were 'The most ghoulish laugh' from the gents and 'The most hair-raising scream' from the ladies. I think the most popular feature was the presence of a fortune-teller, behind a curtain in the corner of the ballroom. The queue (of ladies) would stretch right round the ballroom,

leaving groups of males wondering where their next partner was coming from!

Each summer period there were dancers who for various reasons were spending their holidays at home. It was also a quieter period for us and so we came up with the idea of 'Holidays at home in the Ritz Ballroom'. We discarded our usual band uniform and wore casual seaside clothes to add to the effect. We also placed deck-chairs here and there and erected some 'kiss-me-quick' stalls, besides distributing bars of lettered rock (imported from Blackpool).

The repertoire of a band in those days had to be inexhaustible to deal with all these varied events and one can't help asking oneself how today's 'musicians' might cope. If any multi-millionaire pop idol has wandered into these pages by mistake, he might ask himself the same question.

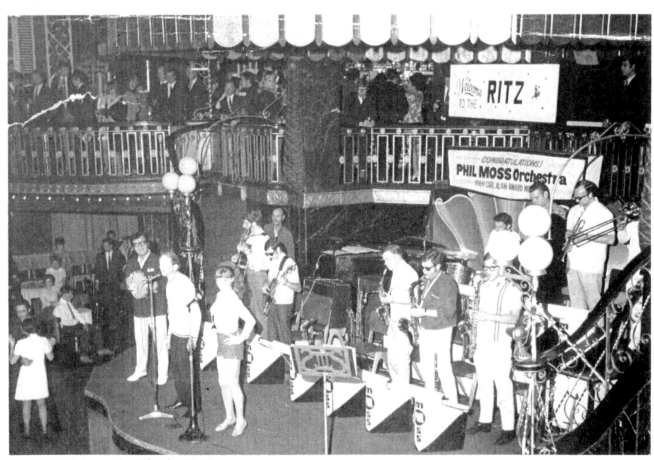

Seaside Night at the Ritz in 1969

Manchester - Home of World Champions

Marcus and Karen Hilton

Had the Manchester area produced world champions in tennis, ice skating or any athletic sport, they would have automatically become household names and instantly recognisable, in the manner of Torvill and Dean. Yet our very own world champions are largely unknown in their own city.

I refer to that very attractive and talented man and wife team from Ashton, Marcus and Karen Hilton, who have won thirteen World Professional Ballroom Dancing titles in all.

They have given dance demonstrations all over the world and attract thousands of admirers abroad. Here in Manchester, I saw them dancing at the Longfield Suite in Prestwich. At one time they were interested in the Latin American dances, but later concentrated on Modern and have for the past five years

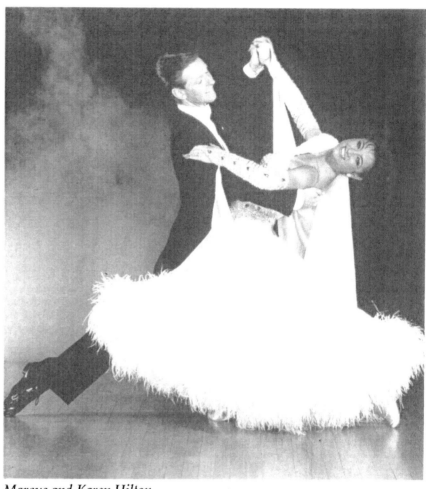

Marcus and Karen Hilton

been the World's Modern Dance Champions.

At the time of writing, ballroom dancing is in the process of being accepted as a sporting event for future Olympic Games. If this does happen, I predict a startling transformation in the local image of Marcus and Karen Hilton.

Bob Dale
Mancunian Star-Maker

When Marcus Hilton was about ten years old he took instruction at Bob Dale's School of Dancing, which was situated next to the School of Music in Albert Square, Manchester. Bob taught there for twenty-two years and he also had schools in Stockport, Levenshulme and

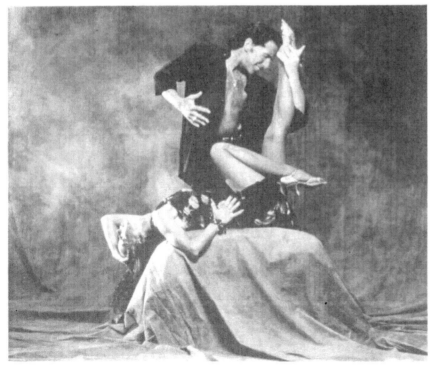

Donnie Burns and Gaynor Fairweather of Manchester, for eleven years World Latin American Dance Champions

Droylsden, which he called the Chalet School of Dancing. For a time he was in the U.S.A, teaching at the Fred Astaire School of Dancing.

The name Bob Dale is synonymous with top-ranking dance events at all levels of the profession. His famous Latin American formation dance team, which he formed and coached from scratch, was consistently successful in the 'Come Dancing' television series. In addition to representing the North West team, from time to time his services were called upon by other regions in the contest.

Perhaps Bob's biggest achievements were in using his coaching talents and some of the most glamorous names in the world of ballroom dancing - such as Marcus and Karen Hilton and Sammy Stopford - owe something to his influence

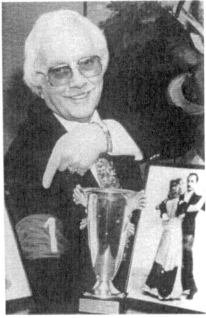

Tommy Moss

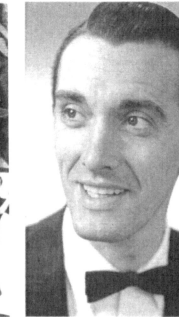

Bob Dale

in the early days of their careers.

Throughout his successful career, which necessitated endless journeys, Bob never considered leaving his

Manchester habitat and he must rank as one of our leading lights in the light fantastic.

Tommy Moss

Before many of the young, present-day champions of the North were born, Tommy Moss was one of those who laid the foundations of ballroom dancing as we know it today. A former World Professional Champion (L'Olympia, Paris) and six times North of England Open Champion, Tommy has taught thousands of people to dance during his long career and he still has a passion for his calling.

Although the Tommy Moss School of Dancing was in his native Wigan, he adjudicated and demonstrated at the Ritz Ballroom, and I also saw him dance at the Astoria Ballroom in Plymouth Grove, Manchester. His own dance school was noted for the presence of his mother, who was widely known as Madame Moss.

Now in his late seventies, Tommy is still a familiar figure in Manchester dancing circles and with his sister Hilda as partner he continues to dance, teach and adjudicate as if it all started yesterday. He enjoys the respect and liking of his

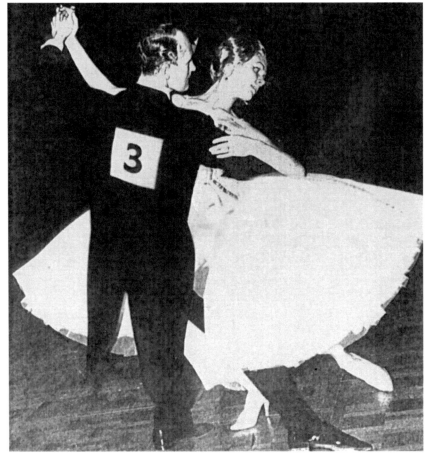

George Coad and Patricia Thompson, former British, European and World Champions

contemporaries and says he will never retire - he hopes his end will take place on the ballroom floor!

Sammy Stopford and Barbara McColl

Sammy Stopford and Barbara McColl became the British, European and U.S.A Open Latin American Dance Champions and I had the pleasure of accompanying them when they gave a brilliant exhibition of Latin American dancing at Kendal's store in Deansgate. When we met I was surprised to find Sammy was much smaller than I had imagined from his television appearances, but he more than made up for any shortcomings with a display of Latin American dances that had the audiences standing up and clamouring for more.

Before the exhibition began I asked him for his preferences and he just said, 'You do the playing, Phil - we'll take care of the dancing.' He had the confidence of a true champion, and it showed.

Sammy lived in Clayton, opened a dance school in neighbouring Droylsden and then one in Stockport. He provided training for all grades of dancers and also travelled the country to give lectures, coaching and exhibitions.

Sammy and Barbara now travel the world and are in great demand abroad, but he will always be remembered as 'Sammy from Clayton, Manchester'.

Pat and George Coad

During my band's many years at the Ritz Ballroom we had the pleasure of accompanying the North West team in all of its inter-regional competitions in the 'Come Dancing' television show. The North West first won the contest about 1956 and won several times after that, as well as reaching the finals quite often.

It would be impossible to catalogue every individual dancer who took part in all those events, but mention must be made of Pat and George Coad, who were ever-present and outstanding in their presentation of the opening event, the Quickstep. I don't recall them ever losing to their counterparts in opposing teams.

There were several sections in the contests, the five modern sections being the Quickstep, Foxtrot, Waltz, Tango and Viennese Waltz. These were followed by the basic five Latin American dances - the Rhumba, Cha-cha-cha, Samba, Paso Doblé and the Jive, which by then had been accepted by the Board as a competition dance. Next was the 'Olde Tyme', then the Off-Beat section (for originality) and finally always the spectacular formation teams.

Pat and George Coad invariably started the first event with their expertise and confidence acting as a spur to the rest of the Manchester team - always roared on by the enthusiastic applause and appreciation of the Ritz Ballroom supporters. George didn't bother to wear the customary competitor's smile, but he looked and acted like a born winner in every other department. With each step he

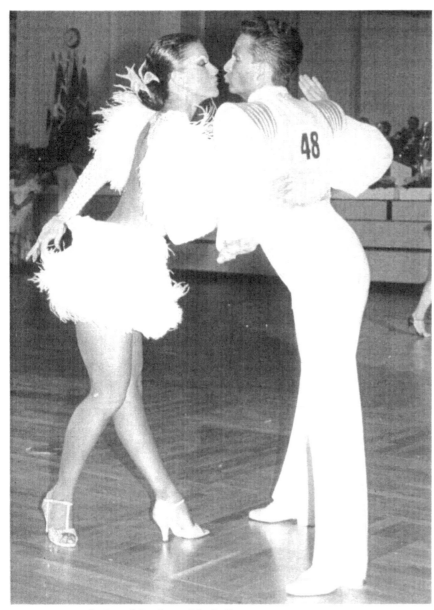

Sammy Stopford and Barbara McColl

exuded confidence and determination. Pat Coad, in contrast, always wore a gracious smile, was willowy and graceful, and ornamental in the extreme. A perfect example of the English rose.

Olde Tyme Dancing - the Mancunian Way

England is known as the Old Country and one of the most popular pastimes in the Old Country was old-time dancing, especially in Manchester and the North West. When the B.B.C's 'Come Dancing' was introduced it always included an old-time section, in which the British Amateur Champions Derek Young and Sheila Buckley were featured. At seventeen years of age they were the youngest couple to win this title and later on (in 1964, 1965 and 1966) they became the British Professional Olde Tyme Champions and Carl-Alan Award winners in 1967.

Whilst on the topic of inventors in the world of ballroom dancing, I must also mention Mr Arthur Dawson from Moston Lane. I can't remember a single occasion in my seventeen years at the Ritz when dance contests were not graced by his

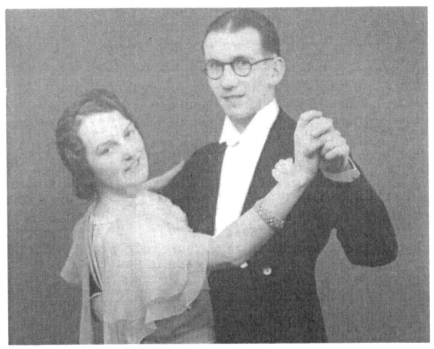

Edith Kershaw and her husband, Arthur Dawson, proprietors of the New Moston Dancing Academy

presence. Arthur Dawson, scrutineer extraordinaire, invented the intricate but accurate system of working out the marks given to each competing dance couple by several adjudicators, in the minimum space of time.

His system was known as the 'Skating System' and it was adopted world-wide. Strangely enough, considering the name,

the system was never used in skating contests. But the world of ballroom dancing owes much to the unique system invented by Manchester's own Arthur Dawson.

Bill and Bobbie Irvine

Bill and Bobbie Irvine were frequent demonstrators on our TV shows at the Ritz Ballroom and whenever they demonstrated the Tango they

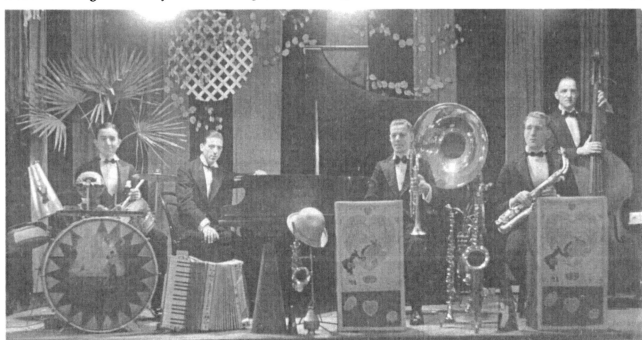

The New Moston Dancing Academy Dance Band

would insist on the band playing 'La Comparsita'. The tune was so hackneyed that we often tried to suggest an alternative, but they were adamant on the subject and invariably won the day - being the World Champions of the day!

Although their origins were oceans apart, Bill hailing from Scotland and Bobbie from South Africa, they gave the impression of being just one person when they were performing on the ballroom floor. During the fifties and sixties they were the undisputed King and Queen of the Ballroom and their successes in championships became almost a formality.

Always friendly and courteous, Bill and Bobbie were the prototype for all aspiring champions and though they have now retired from competitive dancing, they continue to grace the events as adjudicators. They told me that whenever they managed to pay a visit to Bobbie's home town in South Africa they were always

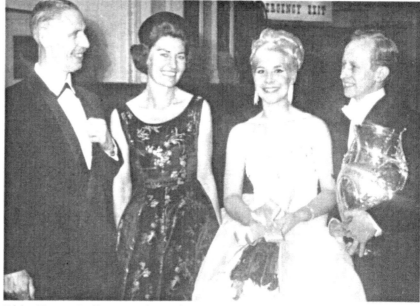

Olde Tyme Ballroom Champions Derek Young and Sheila Buckley (right) with previous winners Alf Halford and Marjorie Robinson. Alf and Marjorie were the inventors of the Lilac Waltz, which has a regular place in dance programmes

reminded of my band - the main store there was called the Phil Moss Store!

Norman and Ada Hilton

Whilst the professional champions make the headlines, the ballroom industry owes much to the thousands of enthusiastic amateur dancers, such as Norman and Ada Hilton, who have been the life-blood of dancing through succeeding decades.

Ada originally took instruction at Finnigan's Dance Academy, but met Norman at the C.I.S. Ballroom in Corporation Street, Manchester. (The C.I.S. was one of the last bastions of Manchester dancing circles and when it closed in 1995 it was a sad day for the dancers who had supported it for many years.)

Ada and Norman formed a team both in dancing and in marriage, winning their many trophies in competitions in Manchester and Birmingham. Eventually they were engaged to give dance instruction and demonstrations on the cruise liner Oceanos.

In the field of dance competition there are far more losers than winners, and as Norman points out, if it weren't for those competitors who persist in their efforts, dance contests would have gone out of existence years ago.

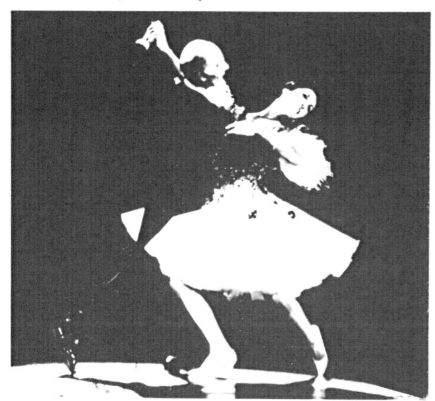

Bill and Bobbie Irvine

The Ritz Revisited

The Ritz Ballroom opened on Whitworth Street West in the twenties and its first patrons were each given a farthing coin, set in a metal base bearing the slogan, 'Keep me, and you will never be broke!'

During the war years the Ritz was swarming with off-duty American G.I.s and uniformed men of all Allied nations and it was hardly surprising that the ballroom became known as the forty-ninth state of America! On weekend evenings Whitworth Street was chock-a-block with jeeps, but the Ritz doormen always reserved a parking space outside the entrance for one jeep in particular, manned by four beefy American service policemen. They were there to watch for undisciplined or incorrectly dressed G.I.s and with their steel helmets, red 'M.P.' armbands, holstered revolvers and batons prominently displayed, they resembled a miniature arsenal for Uncle Sam. If there were any skirmishes involving American servicemen, the M.P.s would wade in and strategic baton blows to the biceps and calves quickly reduced offenders to quivering jelly. Despite appearances, some of these men did have a sense of humour - on the back of one of the M.P.'s vehicles was a hand-made notice: 'Drive carefully. That child in the road could be yours'!

Whitworth Street was thronged with Yankee Doodle Dandies who would saunter down from the Oxford and Palace Bars, wreathed in cigar smoke and with a doll on each arm. The lassies had come from all corners of Lancashire and Yorkshire to see the Stars and Stripes in real life. They had been fed on a diet of Hollywood movies for years and now they had the chance to spot a real life John Wayne, or at least the odd Humphrey Bogart.

Mancunians had little with which to compete in the glamour stakes, but they came into their own when the air-raid sirens sounded. They had been hearing them since September 1939 and the sirens had become about as effective as our car and house alarms are today. It was different with the dough-boys, who had only entered the arena in late 1942. They bolted into the nearest air-raid shelters as per their training instructions, leaving the local heroes in solitary possession of the ballroom until the 'All Clear'. Even the stone image of Abraham Lincoln might have blushed!

It wasn't surprising to see the ballroom heaving with future G.I. brides. The lowliest ranked G.I. resembled an officer in his service dress, and his rate of pay made the British private a second class citizen, to put it mildly. The impressionable girls flocked to the scene in droves and a great many became G.I. brides. A lot came back, too, after the war, disillusioned by the non-appearance of that fabulous ranch and a host more castles in the sky.

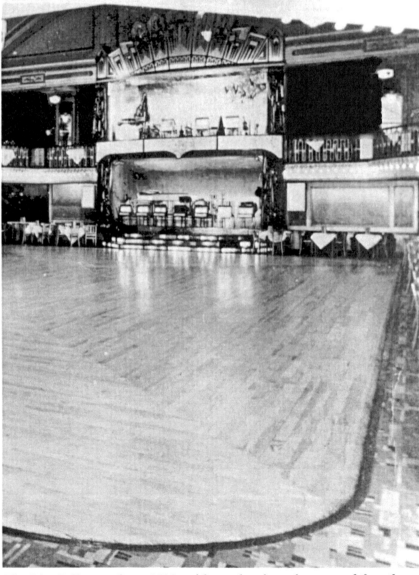

The Ritz Ballroom about 1930, with one bandstand on top of the other

The popularity of the Ritz continued in the fifties and sixties, when it was reported that the ballroom frequently boasted record attendances of over 3,000. During that period, dare I say it, the patrons danced to the Phil Moss Band and Singers!

My favourite slogan in the ballroom was 'Dancing keeps you fit, gentlemen! And it keeps you slim, ladies!' Ballroom dancing presented a pleasant alternative to jogging up a deserted road in the rain, with the odd dog yapping at your heels. The comforts of the ballroom, with its music and friendships, seemed much more inviting and, once inside, all was poise, grace and elegance.

It is said that marriages are made in heaven, but as far as I was concerned they were made on the ballroom floor and I did everything possible to foster romance. I dreamed up the 'Dating Dance', during which I asked people to make a date - at our ballroom, of course! - and played many 'ladies' excuse me', 'gents' excuse me' and even 'general excuse me' dances to keep the mass of patrons well shuffled and to eliminate any 'wallflowers'. We went a step further and introduced the 'kissing arch', mentioned earlier. So many people have told me of their feeling of being in another world when dancing and I have noted a confidence and ability to communicate in dancers which is not given easily to all and sundry.

The Ritz was near the Registry Office in All Saints and so we invited couples who were married around midday to hold their receptions there between 3.00pm and 6.00pm. They could dance romantically under the 5,000 dancing coloured lights in the ceiling (then a big talking point in the ballroom) without paying the high cost of

hiring a hall, and two professional bands played non-stop throughout the afternoon session. We provided a wedding cake if required. Apart from the cost of this, plus admission and refreshment fees, all the rest was free, gratis and for nothing. (Budding entrepreneurs, take note!)

In the fifties the Ritz was closed to the public for two or three weeks whilst the place was given a face-lift and as the company was loath to pay the

contracted Phil Moss Band their wages for being idle during this period, we were dispatched to the Plaza on Oxford Street for the duration.

Now, many girls in those days were warned by their mothers, 'Don't you dare go near that den of iniquity, the Ritz! You can go to the Plaza, but not the Ritz!' Just what the distinction was between the two ballrooms, I never knew. Maybe the Ritz had a reputation because St Mary's Maternity Hospital was

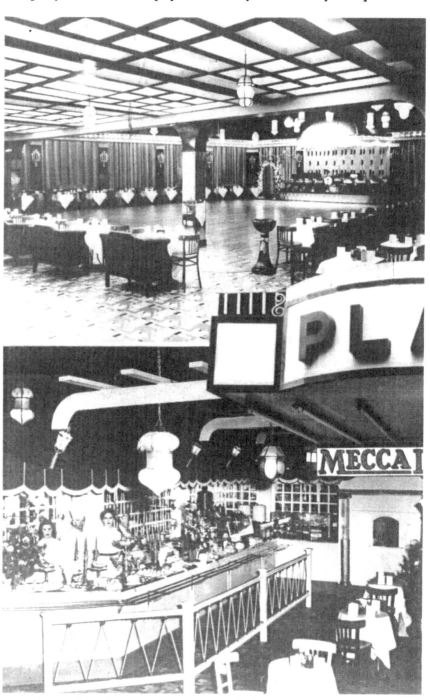

Two views of the Plaza Ballroom on Oxford Street

right next door - it used to be said that the ballroom supplied the hospital with most of its visitors!

Considering the fact that the Ritz was open six afternoons and six nights a week for so many years, it is not surprising that tens of thousands met their marriage partners at the place. One Wednesday in June 1995 I received a telephone call from a Mr Frank Hodges, who asked if it was possible for us to meet that afternoon at the Ritz, where the usual tea-dance still takes place.

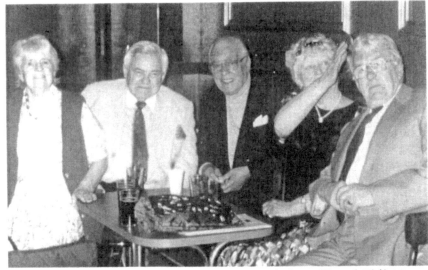

Doris and Frank Hodges (right) with Iris and Jim Gill and Phil Moss (centre)

He and his wife met at the ballroom under very singular circumstances. On 15th March 1948, on a last fling before emigrating to Montreal, Canada, Frank stood on the corner of Whitworth Street and Oxford Street and tossed a coin. 'Heads' the Plaza Ballroom and 'tails' the Ritz. It came down tails. He went into the Ritz at 9.00pm and saw his future wife for the first time. She was then Miss Doris Faulkner. Frank invited Doris to dance and she accepted.

Before the dance finished he had proposed to her on the ballroom floor. She said yes and they have had forty-eight years of happily married life in Canada, with three children and two grandsons.

Others will have their own memories, but Frank and Doris's story is quite unique and on that Wednesday in June 1995 I sat with them at the Ritz, enjoying their obvious delight in reliving their first meeting all those years ago.

I was surprised to see that the Ritz is no longer owned by Mecca, but by the Rank Organisation. The Vic Lazel Band is still playing there and has enjoyed a record stay of twenty or more years.

The Party Spirit

Quite recently a friend asked me to play at his wedding anniversary dance. He said that what he required was the 'party spirit'.

'No problem,' I said. It wasn't until I had replaced the telephone that I started to doubt my optimism. Party spirit is not an article to be bought over the counter - it has to be pursued and it is very elusive, like catching a smoke ring. It is quite possible for a lively trio, playing the party dances of yesteryear, to create a party spirit. It is also possible to

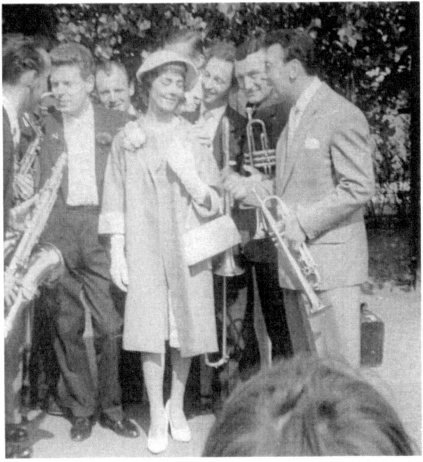

Phil Moss with Mr and Mrs Brown after their All Saints wedding

present a twenty-piece band which is musically perfect, but which is so engrossed in producing that quality that the dancers' needs are in second place.

The serious competitive dancer has two obsessions - the tempo of the music provided and the state of the floor, which can be too slow or too quick, according to how it was polished last. The party spirit is far too frivolous and unimportant to become a consideration for the serious dancer.

The social dancer, however, is critical of other basics, such as the general comfort of the venue, the quality of sundry services and, more importantly, the availability of dance partners. For social dancers, the party dances were a source of variety and pleasure, after the usual Foxtrots and Quicksteps had been accomplished. There was the Boomps-a-Daisy - one of the repetitive movements being a bump on the backside by your partner - to guffaws of laughter.

There was the Hokey-Cokey, with the dancers putting their arms/legs in, out, etc, according

to the bandleader's instructions. Then we had the St Bernard's Waltz, with the dancers stamping their feet on the floor in the fourth bar of each sixteen-bar sequence. Nobody could resist the Conga, formed by a long, continuous line of dancers with a leader weaving all round the ballroom, the tables and even the upstairs balcony.

The Lambeth Walk was another sure-fire winner, with the Cockney words of 'Any time you're Lambeth way - You'll find them all - Doing the Lambeth Walk - Oi!' The Chestnut Tree was another favourite, with the crowd singing and doing the expressive tree branch movements. The Charleston, a throw-back from the twenties, was a good atmosphere dance, energetic but simple, and another survivor was the Gay Gordons, which was a certain rouser when all else failed.

The oldest party dance in my memory was the Paul Jones, the ice-breaker at all functions. All the ladies formed a circle and danced in one direction, while the males formed an outer circle, dancing around the

ladies in the opposite direction - nearly always to the march, 'Here We Go Gathering Nuts in May'. When the music stopped abruptly, each gent would partner the opposite lady and dance to whatever the band played until the march tune started again and the whole process was repeated.

The Progressive Barn Dance was a firm favourite, being a successful crowd mixer, which reminds me of the occasion when my band was playing at Manchester Town Hall at a ball to honour the visit by the Danish Royal Family. The ballroom was packed with all the civic dignitaries and their wives, who could be seen admiring the figure of the Danish Prince, resplendent in his service uniform, which was plastered with medals and insignia.

As he danced past with his partner, other couples gave him a wide berth, until I stopped the music and announced the Progressive Barn Dance. The Prince had the choice of ungraciously leaving the floor or joining in, which he did, to generous applause. In this dance, couples had to interchange progressively, so it gave all the ladies the unforgettable experience of a dance with the Prince. As I looked round the room I could see the paintings of all Manchester's ex-mayors on the walls and they seemed to be glaring down at me with disapproval!

There were many more party dances over the years of ballroom dancing and they gave endless pleasure to generations of dancers. But they are mainly in the past, replaced by excessive noise from the stage, and my friend's request for 'party spirit' at his coming function presented me with a problem. I'm going to put my trust in the old adage, 'It'll be all right on the night'.

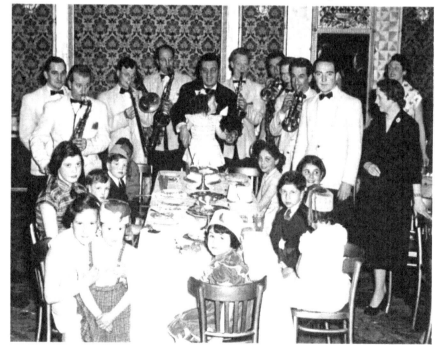

A typical birthday party at the Ritz in 1955

'There is Nothing Like a Dame'

I think it is true to say that if a bandleader added an extra musician to his line-up, hardly anyone would spot the difference. But if he added a young lady vocalist the band would be transformed. World famous film stars such as Betty Grable, Dorothy Lamour and Doris Day started their careers as dance band singers - known in America as 'nightingales', 'wrens', 'thrushes' and 'canaries'.

In general, ballroom dancers disliked dancing to the sound of vocalists and I tried to instil into all my singers the need to sing as near to the actual beat as possible, without compromising their talents. The singers naturally enjoyed singing their own favourites, but again I had to stress the importance of performing those numbers that were currently favoured by Joe Public. Our Joe was a hard taskmaster and it was fatal to lag behind him, or to get too far in front. It was the smart thing to do to keep nicely in step with him. The sweet ballad style of singing was gradually being replaced by a more aggressive style, but by and large we managed to compromise and cope.

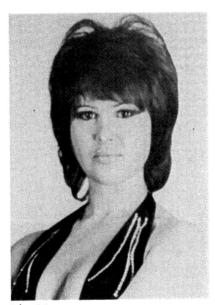

Lisa Young

I was a bandleader for forty years, so I would be hard put to remember every young girl who sang with my outfit, but here are some who will be remembered by the dancers of the Ritz Ballroom.

Toni Sharpe

I will mention Miss Toni Sharpe first, because one participant in our first discussion was unusual, to put it mildly. During the years my band played opposite the Ivy Benson Band at the Villa Marina, Isle of Man, Ivy featured the attractive and talented Toni Sharpe. She was earning a big reputation not only for her singing (à la Ella Fitzgerald), but also for her whistling of birdsong, which was so lifelike that it was said she had the seagulls flying in all the wrong directions!

In view of her growing reputation, I was surprised when she approached me for a job in my band, which was returning to the Ritz in Manchester at the end of the summer season. We discussed the pros and cons whilst sitting in her bed-sit. Toni told me that her Indian guide, 'Broken Wing', had advised her against accompanying Ivy Benson on her forthcoming trip to Russia. I just stared at her - she had to be kidding - but she wasn't. She was into spiritualism and the Indian guide obviously had a starring role in her decision-making.

I had a look round the room. There wasn't a whiff of smoke signals and not even the odd feather floating about. Toni must have read my thoughts and assured me that Broken Wing wouldn't materialise with strangers around. Not that I would have been bothered - any spirit, real or otherwise, that could influence her into joining me was an old friend of the family.

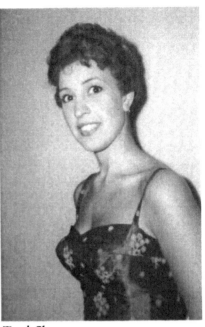

Toni Sharpe

We agreed on terms and the date of starting, which I subsequently posted to the Ritz Ballroom management for advance publicity. So I was shocked some weeks later when Toni announced that Broken Wing had gone through a change of heart and she would not now be joining me as arranged. I had an idea that somebody must have beefed up the Indian guide's commission. Whatever the reason, it was obvious that Broken Wing was now working overtime with the forked tongue and all brotherly love died on the spot. Had he been accessible, his broken wing would have been the least of his worries.

Strangely enough, Toni did in fact join me about a year later, after having married saxophonist Harry Perry. I never heard any further mention of Broken Wing and Toni became a notable asset to my band for a very long time.

Lisa Young

Toni Sharpe was well overdue in her début with my outfit, but Lisa Young booked her appearance years in advance! I'll let her tell her own story: 'It seems to me that many young people nowadays have no idea what they want to do with their lives, even at eighteen years of age. In my own case, I had no such problem. Whilst very young, my mother had taken me to the Ritz Ballroom, Manchester, to watch and listen to the Phil Moss Band and Singers.'

'I had always fancied the music business for my future, and this first visit was enough to convince me that I was to become a professional singer. Once I had made up my mind, we visited the Ritz on many occasions, both of us fascinated by the fourteen-piece band and the thousands of twinkling lights in the ballroom ceiling.'

'At the age of eighteen my dream came true and I became the lead female vocalist with the Phil Moss Band, an association which was to last for many years. To cement my relationship with the music business I went as far as marrying the first tenor saxophonist in the band, Gerry Grant.'

Lisa Young was a pretty young lady, petite in every direction except for her voice, which was powerful enough for someone twice her size. Gerry, Lisa and daughter Amy now have their own band, the Gee-Lees.

Celia Nicholls

My very first lady vocalist was Celia Nicholls in 1950 and many people still remember her singing our theme tune, 'Dancing in the Dark', at the High Street Baths Ballroom. She was everybody's notion of the original 'bonnie lassie' and her Scottish nationality couldn't have been more evident had she walked into that first rehearsal dressed in full Highland kit, playing the bagpipes and singing 'I Belong to Glasgow'! Celia had been regularly featured in radio broadcasts with the Scottish Variety Orchestra, not that this was evident in her singing voice. (What is there in singing that makes all other accents sound English? And eliminates stutters?)

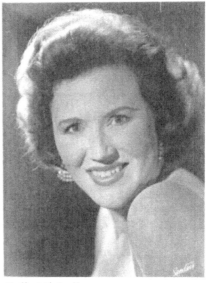

Celia Nicholls

There was something about Celia that radiated warmth. She was quite beautiful, immaculately dressed, thoroughly professional, with a great stage presence and a singing voice to match - probably my greatest single asset in the launching of my first band. She proved a hard act to follow and when she finally left me to join her bandleading husband Ronnie Caryl, she left a

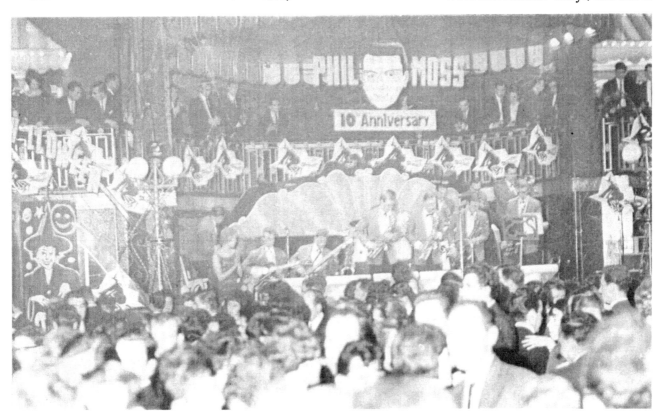

When Ballroom was King. Both the downstairs floor and the balcony are crowded to capacity for the tenth anniversary of the Phil Moss Band at the Ritz in 1964

gap like the Grand Canyon. For many years they were together on the Queen Elizabeth II liner, working with many famous American musicians and bandleaders in the process. Happily, they are still a team, Celia singing as well as ever and Ronnie still turning out his modern arrangements.

Chris Marlowe

There can't be many ballroom dancers of the fifties and sixties who don't remember Chris Marlowe singing with my band at the Ritz and on our broadcasts from the Playhouse. I have a clear recollection of my first meeting with Chris. She bounded into my dressing room and announced that she had just heard I was looking for a new lady singer. She managed to make it sound as if that was all the information she needed

and that I was to be her next bandleader! She was confident, resourceful and had a king-size personality which made that first meeting with the Marlowe seem more like a minor collision.

During my talks on music I have often been asked why some singers reach the top and others of equal ability never get past first base. A smart agent is very often the answer. A smart agent has a talent for using other people's talents and providing he is making a bomb out of it, he'll make sure you are constantly working, like it or not. Chris Marlowe was one of those individuals who didn't seem to need any help from anybody; she had self-confidence and ability in spades. Just put her with a modest trio or quartet and you

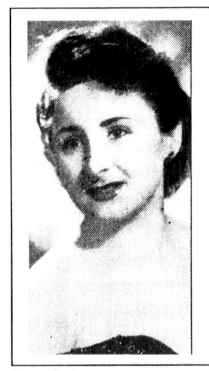

Terry da Costa

had yourself a twenty-piece band on the stage!

Thirty years on since my first meeting with Chris, she still performs like a two-year-old and is still a property to contend with.

Terry da Costa

When I first heard mention of singer Terry da Costa, I thought the name must have been pinched from some brand of cigar, but in fact that was her real name and she had all the equipment necessary to make a fine band singer.

She was one of the few singers who had two distinct voices - one was for dealing with the ballads and the other was a straight soprano - and in the press she became known as 'The voice with a caress.' Terry was quite tiny and once confessed that she always felt lonely sitting on the stage. This was slap in the middle of a large band, surrounded by hundreds of dancers! If I was asked to describe Terry da Costa in a word, I would choose the word 'sweet'. It wouldn't flatter the lady.

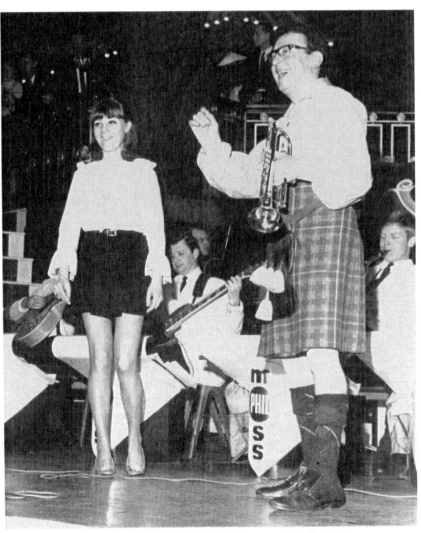

Burns Night at the Ritz with Chris Marlowe and Phil McMoss

The Isle of Man-cunians

Before the introduction of cheap package holidays abroad, the dancing public of Manchester would transfer their activities from the Ritz and Belle Vue Ballrooms of their home town to the massive ballrooms of the Isle of Man and Blackpool.

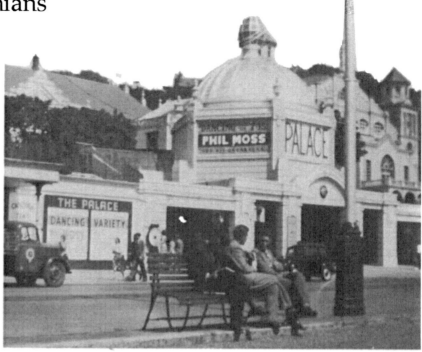

The Palace, Douglas, in 1958

These were the most accessible seaside resorts which boasted some of the largest ballrooms in Europe and presented some of the most famous bands in the country. I had eleven summer seasons at the Villa Marina, the Palace and the Derby Castle in Douglas, and the sight of thousands of dancers tumbling out of their hotels in swarms and making their way to their chosen ballroom was quite a spectacle. The promenade was awash with the ladies swishing along in their long dresses and their escorts carrying the dance shoes under their arms.

They would turn into the Villa Marina, which had the famous bands of Joe Loss and Ivy Benson, or carry on further to the Palace Theatre or Ballroom,

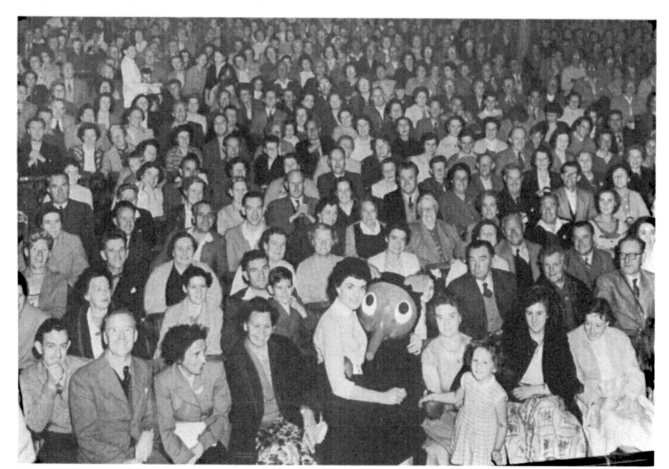

Some of the thousands of Mancunians visiting the Palace Theatre, Douglas, photographed from the stage. Phil Moss vocalist Katrina and Phil's daughter Pamela are at the front

where the renowned Squadronaires awaited them. Further on still was the Derby Castle Theatre and Ballroom, where they could dance to their favourite Manchester band, Phil Moss. During those years, the heyday for big bands and ballrooms, I never tired of waving to hundreds of familiar faces from back home.

The Villa Marina, slap bang in the centre of Douglas Bay, was opened in 1913 and became 'centre-stage' for every top-line artist in Britain. It was indeed rare to meet any Mancunian, anywhere, who had not paid a visit to the 'Villa' at some time or another. The Palace Ballroom was reputedly the largest in Europe, with its spacious gardens and large theatre. The opening night in 1921 was attended by 10,000 dancers and V.I.Ps, plus 3,000 in the gardens - admission 1/6d. The

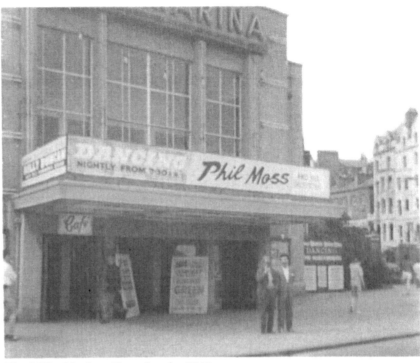

The Villa Marina, Douglas, in 1960

Palace always had an M.C in full evening dress. He would announce the various dances then take up his position in the

centre of the massive floor in order to spot any irregularities. The Palace was the only place in which I played where a three

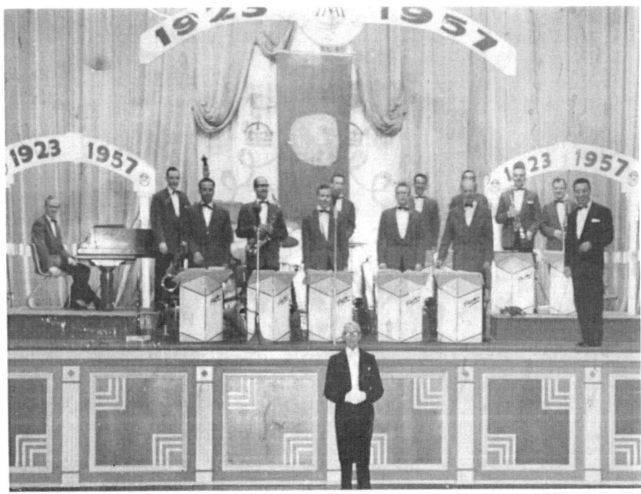

The Phil Moss Band at the Palace, Douglas, in 1957. Note the high stage and immaculate M.C.

minute orchestration would finish before the dancers had negotiated half the floor.

The Derby Castle Ballroom, with its gardens and large theatre, was opened as far back as 1877 and featured famous names of the music hall era - Florrie Forde, George Robey and Vesta Tilley among them. A name familiar today is that of singer Betty Driver (barmaid Betty Turpin on 'Coronation Street'), whom I accompanied in the Derby Castle Theatre in the fifties. Entertainers like Ken Dodd also appeared there early in their careers.

During my seasons at the Isle of Man I tried to match the holiday spirit of the happy visitors by featuring 'singing while dancing'. For this purpose I had slides made containing the words of popular songs of the day and beamed them from a projector on to a white screen on the stage. This proved a winner at the Derby Castle and I used the idea at my daily open-air concerts in the Palace Gardens.

The noise of up to 3,000

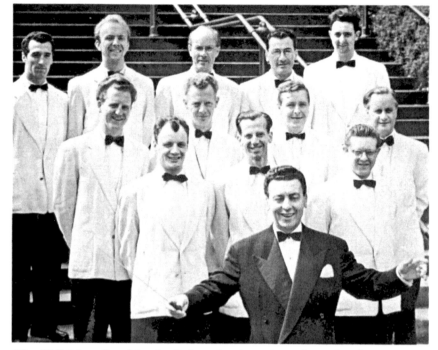

The Phil Moss Band in the Palace Gardens, Douglas, Isle of Man. Back row: Bobby Bell, Derek Tinker, Alf Roberts, Les Moss, Brian Fitzgerald. Middle: Guy Fawkes, Vic Davies, Reggie Winch, Fred Hartley. Front: Ronnie Egan, Johnny Moran, Eric Bennett

holidaymakers singing from their deckchairs was so loud that the more refined music provided by Max Jaffa and his Palm Court Orchestra at the nearby Villa Marina was almost drowned out. The final insult for Max came when the Villa

Marina manager asked him if he could do something similar to what I was doing, in the nature of a fight-back. The notion of asking people to sing 'Ave Maria' and 'Your Tiny Hand is Frozen' outraged the elegant Max Jaffa. His music was impeccable, his audience sat in mute appreciation, while the voices of thousands of happy holidaymakers washed over them relentlessly. Poor old Max didn't appear at the Villa Marina the following season.

There was a similar situation at the Derby Castle, where the ballroom was under the same roof as the theatre and separated by just one door. 'Atty' Baker was the leader of the pit orchestra in the Derby Castle Theatre. He was a diminutive figure and you could just see his head above the pit orchestra rail, but he made up for this by wearing white gloves which flashed in the darkness of the pit.

As a business builder, theatregoers were allowed to leave the theatre and enter the

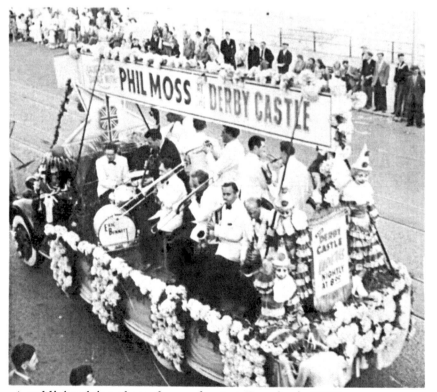

A publicity drive along the sea front at Douglas in 1955

ballroom free of charge, but each time the connecting door was opened, the sound of the larger Phil Moss Band drowned out the music provided by dear old Atty Baker. Often the door would be opened and left open, with disastrous consequences. Once when Ken Dodd was singing 'Tears' on the theatre stage, he swore he didn't know which to follow, Atty's music or mine!

Mancunians have been lured away to take their holidays in other countries since those Isle of Man days, but I'm sure many still remember those horse-drawn tramcars, Manx kippers,

Manx tail-less cats and the immortal song, 'Has anybody here seen Kelly? Kelly from the Isle of Man.'

Personal Glimpses

During the summer seasons at the Villa Marina I had the pleasure of accompanying many famous personalities of the day, such as Diana Dors, Hughie Green, Jimmy Edwards (he of the walrus moustache!), Mike and Bernie Winters and Pearl Carr and Teddy Johnson. They all had, in varying proportions, that common denominator - star quality - and it was interesting to note how each one differed in style and approach. Easily the most nervous of them all was Yana.

Yana

She was one of the most beautiful singers of her day - exquisitely gowned, with a gorgeous figure and a voice which appealed to all age groups. Every reason to inspire confidence in oneself, you might think, yet Yana was the most nervous performer I ever worked with. Just before her first number she beckoned me over in the wings and asked me to feel her heartbeat and it was like somebody pounding on the stage door. She made a hash of

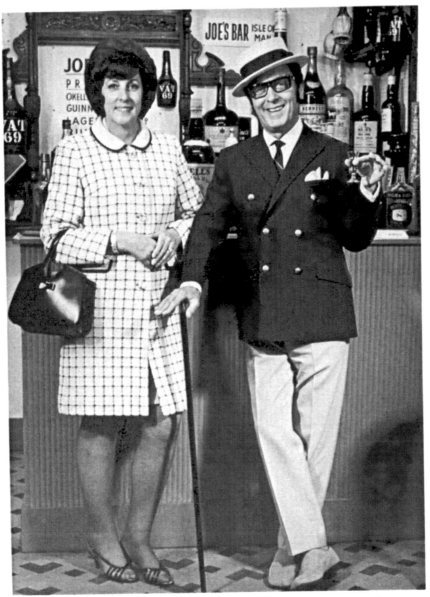

Joan and Phil Moss in Joe's Bar, Strand Street, Douglas. The bar was owned by Alma Cogan's aunt and uncle

the introduction to the opening number, so I cut the band off, started again and this time she rallied round and in the end put on a very convincing show.

Diana Dors

In stark contrast to Yana, Diana Dors was probably the most confident act doing the rounds in 1960. She hadn't the greatest voice in the world, but a total belief in her own ability, together with some knock-out, high-powered American arrangements, made her a convincing package. She was with her husband, Dickie Dawson, and I remember he was surprised at how well my band handled her arrangements. I was more than a little surprised myself!

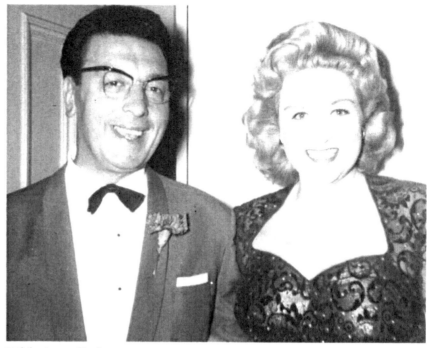

With Anne Shelton

Anne Shelton

When Anne Shelton arrived for band call, she was with her younger sister Jo, also a singer of note. Anne, of course, had been featured with most of the top big bands of the day, including Ambrose and Geraldo. Her approach was entirely different from any of the others. She didn't use the stage much, but had complete composure and a typically English way of singing, which gave her instant rapport with her audiences.

She would have found difficulty competing with today's singers, who depend heavily on energetic movement, but Anne Shelton remains the complete professional in the memory of yesteryear's theatregoers.

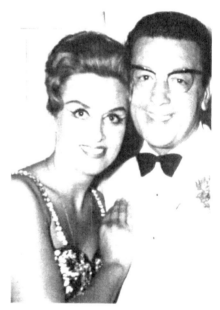

With Yana

Alma Cogan

If you were asked to recall a singer who seemed to have 'the lot', you would probably come up with the name Alma Cogan. She had a bubbling personality, good looks, great presentation and a singing voice second to none in the sixties. She had every requirement for a dazzling career, except good health and sadly she passed away at a very early age. On the occasion she had to cancel her engagement at the Royal Hall in

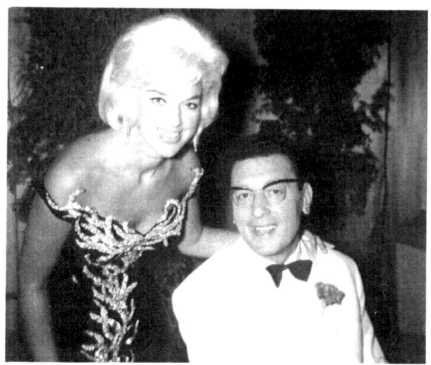

With Diana Dors at the Royal Hall, Douglas

Douglas, a stand-in act was flown over, in the shape of Mike and Bernie Winters.

Mike & Bernie Winters

The brothers made the headlines with their zany comedy in the late fifties. Mike played the clarinet and acted as the straight man to Bernie, who was a naturally funny man - and quite a capable drummer. They complemented each other perfectly and ad-libbed their way through every show. It was a bit of a nightmare for my accompanying band, but at the same time an object lesson in how to clown your way into the hearts of an audience.

Who Pinched the Mayor's Beer?

Playing for public dances, I must admit, isn't always beer and skittles. On one occasion we were engaged to play for the Mayor's Ball at Todmorden and it turned out to be a jolly affair and a night to remember - for more reasons than one.

The Mayor was a smallish, portly figure of a gentleman and he was dutifully followed around by his flock of councillors, with chains of office clanking all over the place. He was lucky enough to win a spot prize, consisting of a small three-bottle pack of beer, which he left on the bandstand for safekeeping.

When the evening came to an end, with back-slapping all round, the members of the band collected their equipment as quickly as possible and off they went in the coach. There hadn't been a cabaret during the dance, but that, as it happened, was due to start. I was the last to leave and during the customary thanks and goodbyes the Mayor popped up, demanding to know the whereabouts of his beer.

We made a search, without any luck, during which the Mayor and his chain gang started to buzz like a swarm of angry bees. The fuss they were making made me suspect that the small bottles were stuffed with state secrets, or at the very least, the Todmorden Crown Jewels.

Knowing my musicians' talents for making beer vanish, I got the feeling that the spot prize had made its way to that great

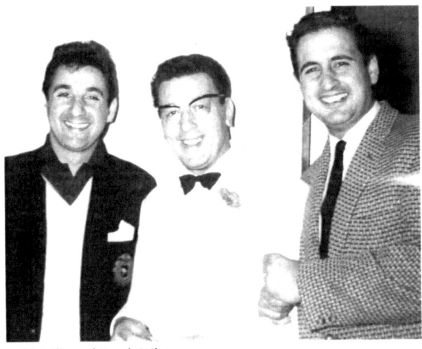

With Mike and Bernie Winters

white brewery in the sky. I could see my new fan club in Toddy vanishing in the same direction, judging by the expressions on the faces of the Mayor's posse. With visions of a possible lynching, I offered to pay for the disappearing ale, but the Mayor scorned the idea and demanded that I make the original pack reappear. Somewhere along the way, he had mixed me up with Tommy Cooper.

By this time I was getting over-excited myself. I asked the Mayor if he thought that I had travelled all that way and knocked myself silly trying to entertain him, just for the real dark purpose of swiping his beer? Not only that, I raged, but I privately hated beer in all its guises, couldn't stand the smell of it and wouldn't touch his spot prize with a ten-foot pole, let alone swig it in secret.

One of the Mayor's chorus said, 'You can't talk to the Mayor like that.' To which I replied that I already had. With that, I tramped out to my car and, just for an encore, slammed the door so hard that it must have shaken the borough's foundations. The last glorious vision I had of our tender farewell was the Mayor surrounded by his retinue, shaking their fists and assuring me that I would never darken their doors again.

Of course, there was a sequel to this story in the shape of a confrontation with my band the following evening. It was then that my lady vocalist (!) admitted she had lifted the nectar in question, thinking it was surplus to requirements. She offered to return payment, which I rejected immediately, demanding she send an exact replica of the pack of beer to the Mayor of Todmorden, saying that it was his original spot prize. As I said, it's not all beer and skittles!

Souvenirs from Blackpool

It wouldn't matter if you were sunbathing in Spain or dancing in Italy. If you happened to hear the strains of 'I do like to be beside the seaside' you would be transported, kicking and screaming, back to dear old Blackpool. To the famous Tower, now over a hundred years old, with Reginald Dixon sitting at the Mighty Wurlitzer again, playing 'that' tune which became synonymous with the Lancashire resort.

You would find yourself wallowing in the nostalgia of the Golden Mile, with its candy floss, tattooed and bearded ladies and 'kiss-me-quick' hats. You would hear the shouting voices of the showmen, inviting you to 'Roll up! Roll up!' and see the fattest lady on earth, or the tallest and smallest men in the world. To view the snake-charmers, hypnotists or the two-headed sea-monster. If you crossed her palm with silver, clairvoyant Gypsy Rose Lee would tell you the colour of

your future husband's eyes, or you could take a peep at the Rector of Stiffkey fasting in a barrel. For a copper coin you could view 'What the butler saw', while the entire spectacle was spiced with the salty aroma of seafood stalls, where cockles and mussels, prawns and shrimps battled with oysters, lobsters and crabs for your attention.

It was all very brash and bawdy, but Blackpool had, and still has, an indefinable vitality that is the envy of the more sedate resorts. Everything about the place was larger than life - seven miles of golden sands stretching from St Annes to Fleetwood; not one, but three giant piers pushing out to sea. Entertainment at every turn, with huge theatres and even bigger ballrooms, attracting some seventeen million visitors every year.

The Opera House, with reputedly the largest stage in

Britain, could seat three thousand people and had the distinction of staging the first Royal Variety Show outside London in 1955.

The famous Big Wheel (the original one) was, like the Tower, a landmark for miles around. Four thousand people queued up to get their first ride, which took up to twenty minutes to complete and it was said you could view five counties from the top. The vast Pleasure Beach was famous for its Big Dipper, which has now been dwarfed by the new highest and fastest roller-coaster ride in the world.

Looking back, Blackpool was a Utopian scene for live entertainment, with bands on all three piers and at the Queens, the Grand, the Palace and Opera House, the A.B.C Theatre, the Winter Gardens and the Tower. It is safe to say that holidaymakers could see a different live show every day of their vacation. Other diversions were available at the Ice Show, the greyhound racing stadium,

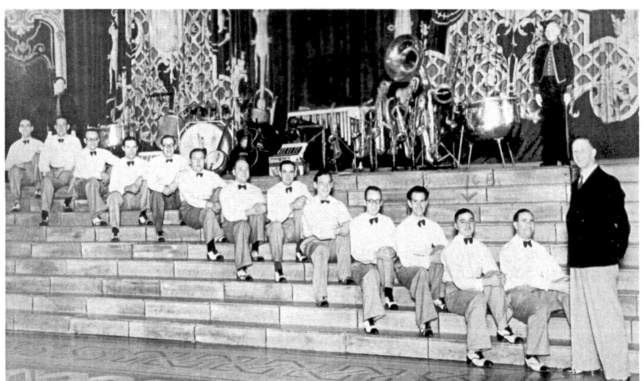

Bertini and his Dance Orchestra at the Tower Ballroom, Blackpool, in 1934. Charlie Barlow is second from right. Note the instruments stacked between the band boys at the rear

boxing and wrestling matches and Louis Tussaud's waxworks museum.

Blackpool had many legendary figures over the years. Bertini and Reggie Dixon at the Tower, Stanley Matthews at the football ground and the great Charlie Cairoli at the Tower Circus. Charlie vowed he would never wear make-up that might frighten children and relied just on his red nose.

There were bands galore, such as Charlie Barlow and his two sons, Ray (guitarist) and Phil (percussion). Freddie Platt (late of the Carlton, Rochdale) was a popular figure, as were Larry Brennan, Tommy Jones, Joe Kirkham and Charles Farrell. Others followed in their wake, such as Ken Turner and Terry Reaney.

My own first season at Blackpool was with Ken Frith at the Burton Ballroom. Mr Bill Hall, then Manchester's leading ballroom entrepreneur, decided to open a hall in thriving Blackpool in 1938 and this was situated over the well known Burton's tailors, right on the sea front at the corner of Church Street. With his usual keen

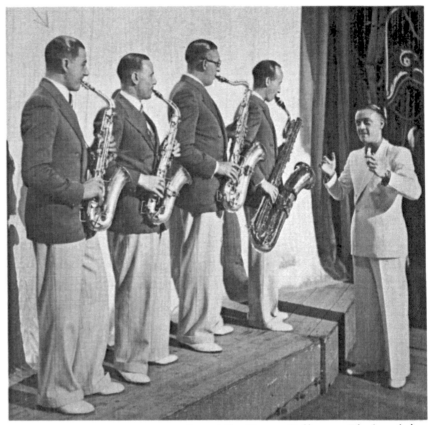

The Norman Newman sax section at the Tower Ballroom, Blackpool, in 1937: Charlie Barlow, Charles Farrell, George Ashwell and Jack Duerden

business acumen, Bill called the place the Burton Ballroom, thus giving the visiting holidaymakers its exact location in the title. Ken Frith, a well-known pianist, was the bandleader and his hand-

picked crew of Manchester musicians proceeded to make a big reputation at the resort.

The Roy Fox Band was at the Palace Theatre when we were at the Burton Ballroom, and their Musicians' Union band steward was Jock Bain. One day he came over to see us with some forms, in order to get us to join the union. This we did, wondering how our boss would react to what seemed to be a step forward for us. Surprisingly, the ballroom manager's mood was quite jovial. He assured us that we had all done the right thing and in future we would be entitled to the full union rate for the job. Our pay would be reduced the following week, as we were getting well over the odds already!

After the war years I did sessions at the Winter Gardens and Tower as a player with the Joe Loss Band. My first

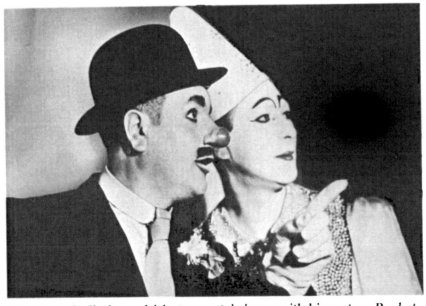

Charlie Cairoli, the multi-instrumental clown, with his partner Paul at the Tower Circus

impression of the Winter Gardens Ballroom was that it was slightly smaller than Grand Central Station but not by a large margin. It was then reputed to be the biggest of its type in the world and was renowned for its parquet floor supported by two thousand springs. The first time I blew my trumpet there, I was convinced that I'd left a mute in the bell!

The Tower Ballroom had much the same effect on me. The Joe Loss Band was a very large one, but we had to spread ourselves out just to give the impression we were really there. It was a paradise for musicians, who in general love to blow their heads off - including myself! It seemed like a ten-minute walk across the stage, but with extra amplification we managed O.K. Later on I led my own band at the Locarno Ballroom and we also played the hotels such as the Imperial, Savoy and Norbreck.

When my band was sent to the Locarno Ballroom we continued to broadcast and play for 'Come Dancing' on television. I

remember for one show, a trombonist arrived in red socks. When I told him it was black socks or nothing, he managed to borrow a pair off the cloakroom attendant!

The music and dance events were synchronised by the floor manager, who was given his instructions from the announcer via headphones. As his arm came down, so my baton would descend, to bring the band in at the same moment as the dancers. I was aided, of course, by my own script which gave the order of events.

Radio programmes were similar, but this time I wore the headphones and the programme started on a red light and finished on a green light. The programme from the Locarno was 'Ray Moore's Saturday Night Out', with the floor packed with holiday dancers. I had to be very alert on those programmes - chatting and joking with Ray Moore in his far away London studio, following the announcements of the Blackpool presenter, conducting the band and

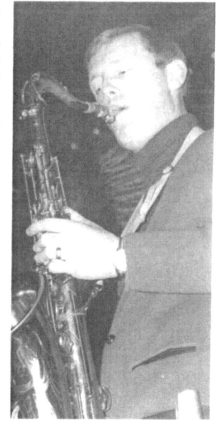

Geoff Lindsay (tenor sax, clarinet, flute) at Blackpool Locarno. Geoff joined the Phil Moss Band at the Ritz in 1958

keeping the ballroom audience happy, and playing for the many thousands of radio listeners. It was all very demanding - but great fun!

Any list of popular bands in Blackpool would have to include the name of Terry Reaney, the successful bandleader and first-class trumpet player with a good singing voice, a flair for showmanship and a very personable image. The first time I saw him was when he was featured in the Ken Mackintosh Band at the Empire Ballroom, Leicester Square, London. Later, he popped up in the David Ede Band at the Locarno in Blackpool and when David Ede was accidentally drowned, Terry eventually took over the leadership of the band, a job he did very successfully.

When my outfit took over at the Locarno in 1970, we did a swap

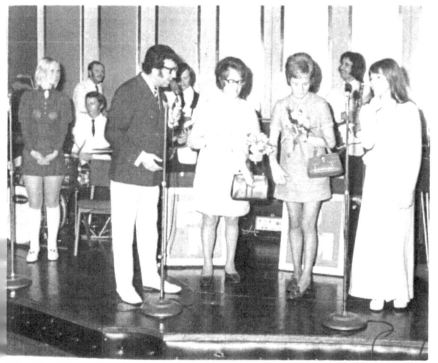

The Phil Moss Band at the Locarno, Blackpool. Singer Chris Marlowe is on the right

and Terry's band went to the Ritz in Manchester. Today, Terry Reaney is a valued member of the Syd Lawrence Band, still enjoying his work and playing better than ever.

The old image of Fred Bloggs with his jugs of tea on Blackpool sands (five shillings deposit in case you legged it with the crockery) has changed somewhat. He was conspicuous then, with handkerchief secured on his head with a knot at each corner, wide braces displayed and paddling heroically with trousers rolled above the knees. But he is still around today, now wearing a baseball cap and carrying a camcorder.

Blackpool has seen many changes over the years, but in some respects hasn't changed at all. The landladies still fry half-a-million eggs and two million rashers of bacon a day during the season. The tonic benefits of the bracing sea breezes are forever free of charge. The various political parties still gather for their conferences. The big dance

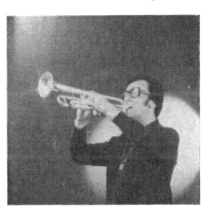

festivals still take place, while the mighty tower, almost six hundred feet high, looks down on the proceedings with a fatherly eye.

Trumpetics

For some reason which I've never fathomed, I've persisted in a life-long ambition to master the art of playing the trumpet. Most people have an ambition of some sort. There are those who want to burrow out of sight in potholes and others who set their sights on climbing Mount Everest, so measured against those, I suppose my own ambition wasn't too unreasonable.

But I must confess right now that I never mastered the instrument in the fullest sense of the word. When my family and colleagues ask how, then, did I manage to play on hundreds of recordings and broadcasts, my answer is, 'With much effort!'

The virtuosos such as Raphael Mendez, 'Doc' Severenson and Harry James made the trumpet an extension of themselves, merging man and instrument into one entity. With me it was always the two of us, with the usual disagreements. Nevertheless, I've always felt a certain pride in the instrument, which has survived all musical trends and instrumentation over the centuries.

Back in the days of the Roman

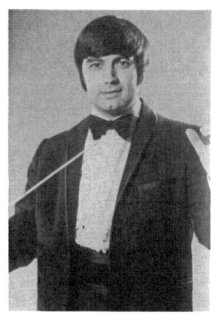

Terry Reaney, trumpeter, vocalist and bandleader

Empire, civic dignitaries were greeted with the fanfare of trumpets. As I write, this week marks the fiftieth anniversary of the end of World War II and we didn't hear guitars twanging at the Cenotaph - just the stirring sounds of trumpets to herald the two minutes' silence for the dead. When the Queen opens Parliament there are no wailing saxophones, but again the impressive fanfare of trumpets. The same trumpets have ordered men into battle and commanded them to retreat.

One kind lady assured me that to play the instrument you just needed plenty of puff. So I blew as forcefully as I could down my own - without producing a squeak. 'Ah,' she said, 'but you didn't twiddle those knobs, did you?' She was referring, of

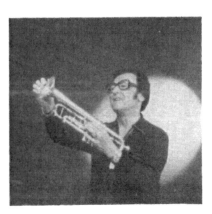

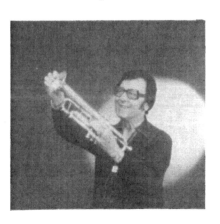

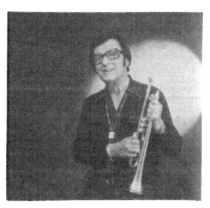

course, to the valves which shorten or lengthen the amount of tubing. So I pressed them all down, singly and together, still without the obliging squeak.

As a matter of interest I must explain that music is created by vibrations. By strings on violins and guitars and by reeds on reed instruments such as saxophones and clarinets. The sounds from trumpets and other brass instruments are created by vibrations on the lips inside the mouthpiece. The trumpet itself is just a length of tubing which amplifies the sounds created by the tension of the lips (or embouchure) inside the smaller mouthpiece. The valves on the instrument are used to shorten or lengthen the amount of tubing required for a particular note; the moving slide on a trombone has the same effect.

This is not a treatise on how to perform on brass instruments, but it should explode a few myths surrounding the trumpet. Should the reader still be confused about vibrations, I recommend taking a comb and

paper and blowing through them. The paper will vibrate against the comb, the vibrations will tickle your lips and you will be able to hum any tune you wish. Voilà! You are a musician without realising it!

The 'Golden Trumpet' (à la Eddie Calvert) was a popular myth. The cost of making such an instrument would be prohibitive and even if one were made it wouldn't have the resonance or carrying power of brass, the metal from which trumpets are made.

A final friendly word of advice to budding players of the trumpet. Providing you have been taught correctly, you are making progress and are happy with that progress, stick to the same method and practise regularly. I mention that in the sincere hope that you won't fall into the trap of changing from one method of playing the trumpet to another, as I did.

Having successfully progressed from amateur to professional status, I made the fatal error of trying to improve on what

nature had intended. I decided to adopt the 'no pressure' method, which entailed suspending the trumpet by a piece of string, so making it virtually impossible to use pressure.

I spent much time on this and then I read about the 'closed lip' method. Next, I read another treatise which insisted that correct breathing was the salient factor in trumpet playing. To effect this I had to place one hand on the diaphragm to check on the correct procedure. This was followed by the 'Buzz' method of creating the lip vibrations, then the 'Pivot' system, which entailed blowing into the top of the mouthpiece for the high tones and the bottom part for the lower tones.

In the end I became a trumpeting hypochondriac, with no recollection of what had made me an adequate and competent player in the first place. I had reached the bizarre stage where I had to seek a band - and bandleader - who would be happy to have me sitting on the stage with my trumpet suspended from above and with one hand resting on my diaphragm. Then sitting bolt upright, neither stretching my lips nor pouting my embouchure, buzzing into the mouthpiece in see-saw fashion, and seeking the perfect method which doesn't exist.

The happy alternative is to play in a natural and comfortable manner which breeds self-confidence. This is an important exercise in itself and confidence is a subject I have yet to see discussed in any tutor book.

Finally, a student who aims for a reputation as 'the player who never misses a note' is reaching for the moon. In practice, it is better to play well within your capabilities in public. They never know your limitations until you expose them.

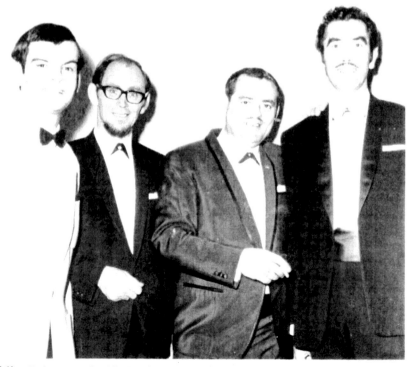

Eddie Calvert, of 'Oh Mein Papa' fame, as a member of the Plaza Band, Stockport

Make Believe Ballroom

Several years ago, right out of the blue, I received a phone call from the studios of Granada Television. Would my band be available to take part in a nostalgic television show at my old stamping ground, the Ritz Ballroom? We certainly would! The show was to feature the Phil Moss Band and an invited crowd of dancers, ex-patrons of the place when it was in its heyday.

Came the evening of the programme, the Ritz was taken over by Granada, the band was assembled, the dancers were at the ready and Anthony Wilson was doing the commentary. We went through a typical programme, with the cameras focused on the dancers and the band, and there were interviews with the old-timers.

When the programme came to an end the band departed (probably to the nearby Palace Bar), the television crews packed up and the last of the dancers drifted out into the darkness of Whitworth Street, leaving just myself and the night-watchman in the building. He was busy making a cup of tea for us both whilst I sat and stared into the shadows of the ballroom and the balcony café, gazing into a thousand memories.

The night watchman went upstairs to check and tidy the offices, giving me the opportunity to wander round the silent ballroom on my own and to keep a date with some old but never-to-be-forgotten ghosts of the past. I thought I could hear a faint scratching near the bandstand - it was probably some music-loving mouse. The revolving bandstand was still, but as I got near it seemed to glide round and there was Charlie Bassett and his trio, grinning and playing the turn-round tune, 'Lovely Lady' - good old Charlie! Then the crimson jackets of my own band came into view. The band brassily took up the melody and there

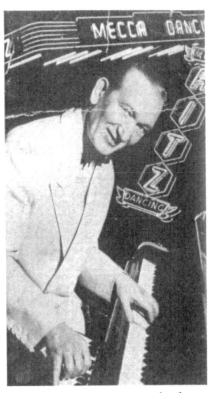

Charlie Bassett, quartet leader to the Phil Moss Band at the Ritz

was the crowd of dancers, gazing up at the changeover expectantly.

Suddenly it was New Year's Eve. There were streamers and balloons galore and the patrons were shaking hands, singing

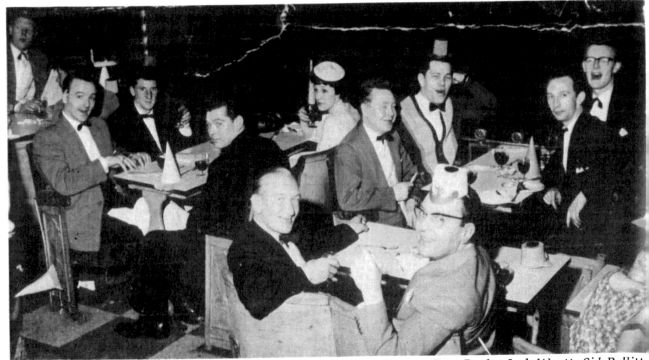

Christmas Eve at the Ritz about 1960. Left to right: Norman Brown, Don Banks, Jack Wyatt, Sid Pollitt, Miss Toni Sharpe, Reg Winch, Pete Brown, Alan Clarkson, Geoff Lindsay. At the front: Charlie Bassett and Phil Moss

'Auld Lang Syne', kicking the old year out and welcoming in the new. Matt Busby and his party were waving me over for a drink; my wife and family were beckoning me to join them. Manager Jack Binks was striding over, his jet-black hair shining like the floor of the Hammersmith Palais, dutifully followed by his assistants, Les Byron and Danny Segal. I could see all my old friends: Colin Rigby of Quicks, Bobby Charlton, Bill Benny, Stuart Hall, and Jimmy Savile over from the Plaza.

But the scene began to fade away and I could now hear another voice, the announcer of 'Come Dancing'. My band was playing the introductory music; George and Pat Coad and the North West team were swirling confidently into the contest with the opposing team. Cameramen were all over the place and hundreds of members of the Manchester audience were roaring their heads off in partisan encouragement.

The scene changed again. The cameras were still busy, but this time they were focused on the faces of Dora Bryan and Rita Tushingham. We were filming the ballroom scenes for the film,

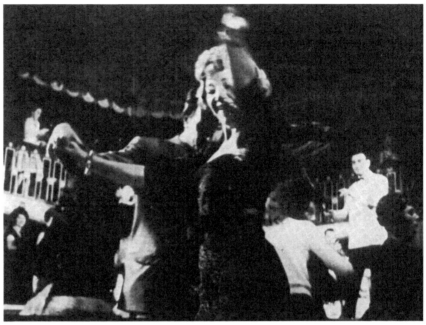

A still from the film 'A Taste of Honey'. Dora Bryan is in the foreground and Phil Moss (white jacket) conducts his band at the Ritz

'A Taste of Honey' and Dora was wearing her usual big grin. Rita Tushingham was slightly apprehensive - it was her first major screen rôle.

There was another change of scene and the Phil Moss Band was again playing for public dancing. It was the last waltz, with a packed floor of dreamy dancers all loath to end the evening and my band was whispering 'I'll See You Again'. I

imagined I could hear Danny Segal urging me to hurry up as he was waiting to lock up. But it wasn't Danny, it was the night-watchman, very real and very much in the flesh, jingling his keys suggestively.

I said thank you and goodnight and went outside to my parked car. I'd had the pleasure of meeting a lot of ghosts that night. I just hope the feeling was mutual.

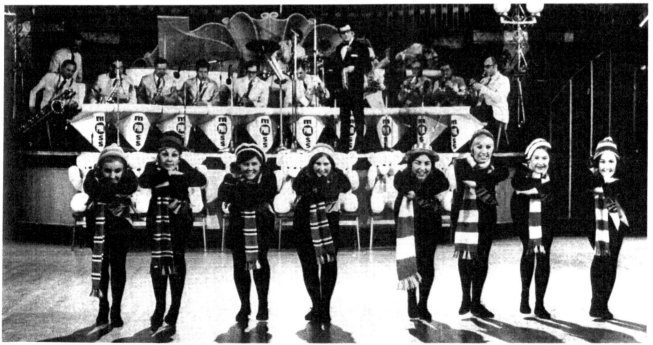

'Come Dancing' at the Ritz - the Off-Beat section

When the Phone Stops Ringing

'When the phone stops ringing' was a phrase I vaguely remember being used by the old-timers in the musical profession. It held no significance for me when I was a young freelance trumpet player: the phone would ring out cheerfully and persistently, acting as my unpaid agent and manager. I progressed to being a very successful lead trumpet player with the Joe Loss Orchestra, then in 1950 I became a bandleader and my staunchest ally, the phone, continued to do its stuff enthusiastically.

Big changes were taking place in the background, with the pop record industry booming and disc jockeys replacing bandleaders - new names, new sounds, and one by one my contemporaries were disappearing from the scene. I was well established and luckier than most, but the number of band engagements was dwindling ominously. The phone was silent for longer, and still longer intervals. Then it became silent - and stayed that way.

My mind was reluctant to accept the obvious. Quite illogically I would check the telephone exchange to see if my phone was out of order. Later I decided to change its location - maybe sunlight would breathe some life into the corpse. I discussed the idea of a new phone with my wife - a brighter colour, perhaps? The look she gave me suggested I might be losing my marbles. In retrospect, I think she could have been right.

I even dreamed about the wretched thing - I was in Telephone House, lost in a sea of offices among thousands of forlorn-looking, discarded telephones, searching for mine, when it suddenly started ringing.

I had been awakened by the sound of the real phone ringing and I went down the stairs two at a time to snatch up the receiver.

'Mr Moss?' came the polite voice.

'Yes!'

'Could you possibly change your dental appointment to later in the day, please?'

'Why, yes,' I said. 'Of course.' Why not? Where the devil did she imagine I might be going anyway? I stared at the phone - it seemed to be grinning at me. It was within an ace of being strangled by its own cord.

There were compensations, of course. That's how Nature works. I was now able to visit my family more often and enjoy the warmth of their affection. New friends materialised and there was the growing realisation that I had been living everyone's life but my own. But I still had the habit of occasionally looking up at the wall clock at the time I would normally start to play.

I was doing precisely that one evening when the front door bell rang. It was Easter Monday and my birthday. My two daughters and five grandchildren trooped in, laden with Easter eggs and singing 'Happy Birthday'. I was suddenly so thankful that I was here, at home, and not away on some God-forsaken one-night stand.

I looked over to the telephone. It seemed to have lost its air of hostility and managed to look quite amiable, in fact. For the first time we were in complete agreement. I realised that in its own inscrutable way, it had been trying to convey a message for a long, long time. That there has to come a day - for all of us - when the phone stops ringing.

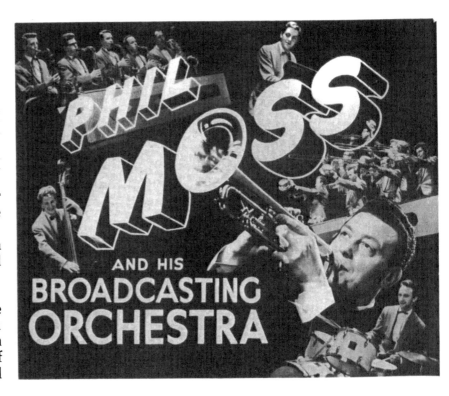